GOOD HANDS

A guide to the techniques and skills that will enable you to give a massage with the confidence, the effectiveness and the touch of an expert.

GOOD HANDS

MASSAGE TECHNIQUES FOR TOTAL HEALTH

ROBERT BAHR

Illustrated by Martin Lemelman

THORSONS PUBLISHING GROUP
Wellingborough * New York

First UK edition 1986

NOTE TO THE READER

The ideas, procedures, and suggestions contained
in this book are not intended as a substitute for consulting
with your physician. All matters regarding your health
require medical supervision.

Published by arrangement with New American Library,
New York, NY.

British Library Cataloguing in Publication Data

Bahr, Robert
  Good hands: massage techniques for total health.
  1. Massage
  I. Title
  615.8'22   RM721

  ISBN 0-7225-1280-5

Printed and bound in Great Britain

To Charles Gerras,
who believed when I needed a believer

CONTENTS

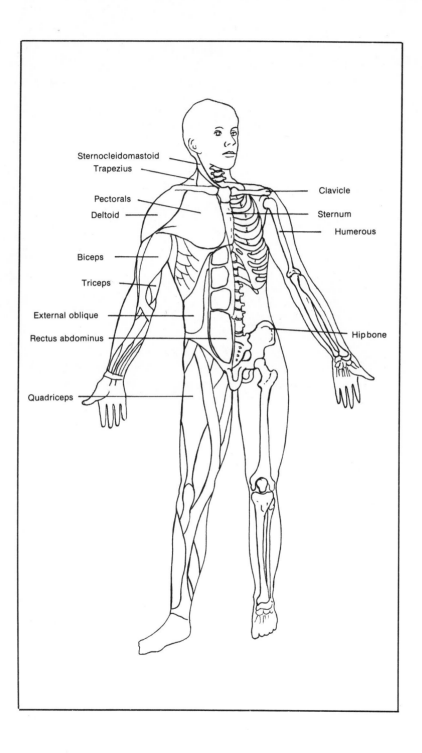

Sternocleidomastoid

Trapezius

Clavicle

Pectorals

Deltoid

Sternum

Humerous

Biceps

Triceps

External oblique

Rectus abdominus

Hip bone

Quadriceps

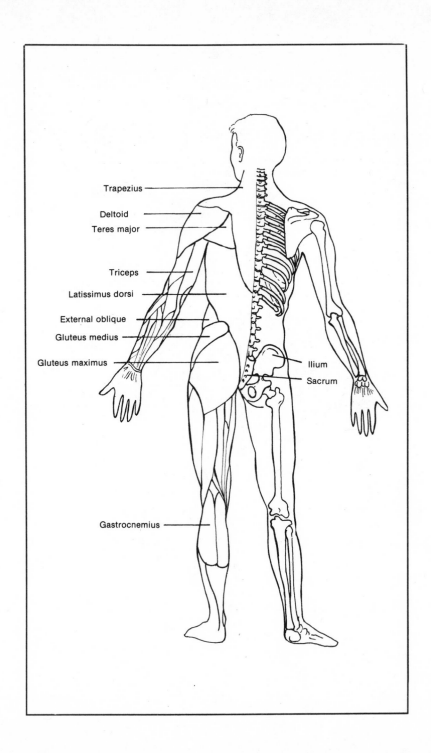

Trapezius

Deltoid

Teres major

Triceps

Latissimus dorsi

External oblique

Gluteus medius

Gluteus maximus

Ilium

Sacrum

Gastrocnemius

PART I
WHAT'S IT ALL ABOUT?

CHAPTER ONE

HOW MASSAGE WORKS

The instant you place your hands on another person's body, things start to happen. Some are emotional, others physical, and they are all good. Sometimes, they border on the miraculous, and as you study this book, they will be miracles you, too, will learn to perform using massage techniques that have been perfected over the ages.

Good Hands will teach you the skills of massage. First, you will learn the techniques of *classical* massage—a whole-body relaxation massage that some people call Swedish, others modern, and others just "strokes." It's the best way to relieve tense, tired or stiff muscles. It improves circulation. It relaxes the tense and stimulates the weary. With specialized classical techniques, you can massage your baby, an elderly or invalid friend, or an athlete. Or you can use massage for beauty—and for lovemaking.

The second type of massage you will learn embraces the techniques commonly called deep friction massage, connective tissue massage, reflexology, and shiatsu. I call it *finger pressure* massage. You will learn how to use it to give relief from a stiff neck, an arthritic shoulder, a cramped thigh, a spasmed or cramped muscle, and many other acute or simply bothersome pains.

We'll start at the very beginning; I won't even assume that you know precisely what massage is right now. My best friend didn't. He returned from a visit to a chiropractor and told me he'd received a wonderful massage. It turned out he hadn't had a massage at all, but an adjustment. Massage isn't bone cracking. It isn't traction, naturopathy, chiropractic, yoga, or modern medicine

—although practitioners of those disciplines might also use massage.

Massage is the manipulation of the body's soft tissues—primarily the muscles: kneading, rubbing, tugging, slapping, hacking, and pressing them to enhance their well-being. A good massage depends on your good hands.

What do I mean by "good hands"?

In the words of masseur Ed Haley of the Holistic Health Center in Allentown, Pennsylvania, "All massage is a science in its psychological effect, but an art in its application." Now that's a crucial point, and I'll be repeating it throughout the book. And if I say it a hundred times it won't be too often: Massage is both a science and an art.

Giving a massage is like playing a violin. With a little talent, you can learn the rules of reading music and the fundamentals of playing the instrument. But to be an artist you must go beyond the rules. You must interpret, allowing the feelings inside you to flow through your fingers, to produce something beyond what is written on the page.

When you give a massage, the flesh beneath your hands will respond to your touch. At first you might detect tension or guilt in resistant flesh that seems to be saying, "You're wasting your time —you must have more important things to do." "It's embarrassing to be made such a fuss over." "I feel so helpless." You'll sense those feelings in the tightness of the muscle, feel them with your fingers. But as the massage continues, you'll sense another message coming through. "That feels good there. You've made those muscles relax. I couldn't do it by myself." "You make me feel important, I'm grateful to you." "You're very special to me for making me feel this way."

You can learn to use your hands with grace and skill, interpreting signs of tension, pain, resistance, and pleasure, and responding in a symphony of effective, coordinated movements.

What Massage Can Do

There's a lot more going on during a good massage than most people realize. In recent years, researchers have begun doing serious studies on the effects produced by massage, and we now know that massage works psychophysiologically, which simply means that it treats both mind and body simultaneously.

When your hands touch a person's skin, the nerves in his or her body awaken immediately. They relay the "touch" message to the brain's switchboard (called the hypothalamus) where the touch is interpreted. The switchboard sends out "reaction" instructions through the nervous system and the hormonal system, and those responses travel throughout the whole body. Massage can stabilize respiration and heart rate, but a single feathery touch in a sensitive area can also start the heart racing, the palms sweating, and produce a drastic change in emotional outlook. A single stroke can increase the body's awareness and sensitivity, induce euphoria, and decrease tension. The effects of massage are varied and frequently dramatic.

Massage improves blood circulation in ways similar to exercise. During exercise, the circulatory system functions at optimum efficiency. Blood vessels dilate, including the tiny capillaries that carry oxygen and other nutrients to the skin and remove the waste products that would otherwise build up. The heart contracts more powerfully to send more blood to these expanded vessels.

As exercising muscles rhythmically contract and relax, they massage the veins, "milking" them, to force the blood back toward the heart. This natural muscle massage is the primary means whereby blood is circulated through the veins. People who don't exercise often suffer pooling of blood in the veins, particularly the legs, which can stretch the vessel walls until they rupture: a condition known as varicose veins.

Like exercise, massage milks the veins. Even the most gentle massage produces immediate capillary dilation—you can see the reddening of the skin and often feel the increase in temperature from the improved blood flow. After a thorough massage, the volume of blood circulating can actually double, as it will with exercise, but one study shows that the blood volume will remain high about four times longer than it will following exercise.

The body responds to the increased blood flow by producing more red blood cells, ones that carry oxygen to every cell in the body. Obviously, increased oxygen supply means increased metabolic capacity and healthier cell functioning.

Increased circulation also means that more wastes are removed from spaces between the muscle tissues where it has accumulated. These wastes—lactic acid and such—can cause the muscular aches and pains we all experience from time to time, and massage, by helping to remove them, can bring relief.

Improved circulation is particularly important in treating sports-related injuries, according to exercise physiologist Dr. Charles T. Kuntzleman. He writes in *The Physical Fitness Encyclopedia:*

The process of recovery from injuries involves the removal of excess fluids that have collected, the actual repair of damaged tissue, and the breakdown and removal of adhesions and destroyed tissue substances. Massage increases circulation in the area of the injury. The blood brought into the area by the increased local circulation provides nutritive, rebuilding materials, and facilitates the removal of the excess fluids and tissue debris from the injury.

Massage also has a dramatic effect on the lymph system, a network similar to the blood circulatory system but consisting of only capillaries and veins. The lymph system absorbs waste and excess proteins from the spaces between body cells and returns them to the bloodstream from which they can be metabolized and excreted; a severe blockage in the lymph system prevents siphoning off of these substances and leads to extreme swelling, the disease known as elephantiasis. The lymph system also traps dust and bacteria and manufactures lymphocytes, which defend the body against infection.

The frog has a marvelous means of moving lymph through the veins to where it pours into the bloodstream: four rhythmically pulsing lymph "hearts." We humans are less fortunate. We have no lymph hearts, and the heart we *do* have isn't connected to the veins and capillaries of the lymph system. Lymph from all over the body oozes through the lymph system to the main lymph vein in the left shoulder, where it finally drains into a vein of the blood system. It's nudged along by nothing more than the massaging motion of your skeletal muscles and the rising and falling motion of your chest as you breathe.

It's obvious why exercise is so important to lymph circulation, but here again, massage produces a similar effect, speeding up lymph flow and clearing blockages in the system that could otherwise cause edema, or swelling. Massage can cure painful swelling of the limbs and other problems caused by a blocked or sluggish lymph system.

That's still just the beginning of what massage can do for the body. Physical therapists have used massage successfully to prevent or reverse muscle shortening and stiffening which occurs when a limb is injured or not sufficiently used, loosen chest congestion when the mucous is too thick to be coughed up, soften scar tissue and make it more flexible, ease the pain and stiffness of certain forms of arthritis and bursitis, and treat insomnia, tension headaches, stress tension, and depression.

The miracle of massage goes beyond its direct physical effects.

When you put your hands on another's body, no matter how clinical the environment, you're touching *emotion* as well as flesh.

"Touch has always been a most effective method of healing," says Bernard Gunther in his book *Sense Relaxation*. "The energy that flows through the hands can refresh, regenerate, revitalize. The laying on of hands can create great physical–mental changes. In the hands of a person who understands, touch sometimes can be as effective as drugs or surgery."

In a series of experiments, James Lynch, professor of psychiatry at the University of Maryland School of Medicine, gave a mild electric shock to the legs of dogs and horses and found that their heart rates increased drastically. Then he repeated the test, this time petting the animals, and found that their heart rates remained normal.

A researcher, Patricia Heidt, found that patients admitted to a hospital with suspected heart attacks became more relaxed after five minutes of casual touching—taking their pulses at four places —than they did when the time was spent simply talking with the nurse.

What Massage Cannot Do

Now, let's discuss what massage *cannot* do. One author has written, "You need no longer live in fear of so-called incurable diseases; nothing is incurable . . . ," implying that anything from cancer to ingrown toenails can be massaged away. Unfortunately, several "schools" of massage are built on this messianic approach. In fact, massage is usually very effective for *certain* conditions, but *no* massage will cure tooth decay or mitral valve prolapse.

It's to be expected that certain massage practitioners should hold a cultlike view of their specialty. Most have theories to support their claims, usually based on the idea that manipulation of the surface blood vessels, lymph system, and nerves has a profound effect on all aspects of the body.

Many people believe such reasoning. I don't say it's impossible, but I *do* say there are no controlled scientific studies to verify the claim that massage can *cure* cancer, heart disease, and other serious organic ailments, although it might help to relieve pain and even *contribute* to the cure, depending on the nature of the illness.

As a wise massage-giver, you need to work *with*, not in place of a trained physician when illness exists.

There *are* times when massage should definitely *not* be used.

- If there's a possibility that a bone has been broken, you could do serious damage to muscle tissue and blood vessels by massaging.
- If a person is unconscious, vigorously massaging the extremities could increase the drop in blood pressure and cause shock.
- Whenever massage causes significant pain it should be discontinued. Pain may signal a severely torn muscle, ligament or tendon, peritonitis, appendicitis, infection, and a host of other ailments that can be made more serious by vigorous massage. Although some types of massage *do* require painful manipulation, practitioners must be carefully trained in the techniques to avoid injury.
- Massage is contraindicated for an inflamed infection from which the infecting bacteria can be spread to other tissue; when bone tissue is the cause of arthritic, rheumatoid, and similar conditions, when serious skin conditions exist, or when there's a possibility of dislodging a blood clot in a blood vessel.

Before massaging anyone with a medical condition, check with a medical doctor to be sure you won't complicate the ailment.

Now you know how massage works: what it can do, what it can't do, and when it should not be used. Massage won't work at all in giving the physical and emotional benefits I mentioned, however, without one key element: the right environment.

The first massage I ever had was at a YMCA health club. My idea was to get the tight muscles in my neck and shoulders softened up so that, after several months of deadline pressures, I might take the first steps toward learning how to relax again.

The masseur knew his stuff. He'd been a full-time professional for more than 20 years. Yet, the massage was useless in helping me to relax, although it wasn't the masseur's fault. The problem was the room—glaring white walls and bright overhead lights.

In the years since that experience, I've come to understand and appreciate the importance of environment to a good massage. Your hands can bring pleasure, ecstasy, relief from pain, and healing— but the place and setting, as well as the time, must be right.

In the next chapter, you'll learn how to create just the right environment.

CHAPTER TWO

THE RIGHT ENVIRONMENT

The Right Place

People give massages for any number of reasons, and there are as many right places as there are reasons. Massage following injury is best given in a well-equipped physical therapy room. You might give sensuous massage in the bedroom or in front of a fireplace. In general, the ideal location for a massage will meet the following criteria:

The right place is a pleasant place to be. Whether indoors or out, you and your friend should feel good about the surroundings—as they say, there should be "good vibes." Indoors, the colors most conducive to relaxation and mutual trust are the soft, warm, neutral ones: beige, ivory, olive, and such. Heavy colors can be stifling, pale colors such as light blue, green, and white can be cold, and shades of red can be threatening and tension-building for some people. Make no mistake: We all react unconsciously to the colors that surround us.

Select the environment most conducive to the type of massage you're giving. A small room encourages intimacy, a medium-sized one friendliness. A large room suggests distance between you and the person you're massaging, and should be used only for therapeutic massage.

Outdoors, space seems to have a different effect. On a private beach, in the woods, a field, garden or backyard, the atmosphere is spontaneous and free, and in my opinion those are ideal locations for close friends to share a whole-body massage. In fact, the best massages I've ever given or received were in a small grassy area near a pond in the woods where I live in northeastern Pennsylvania. On a summer afternoon, with the warm sun filtering through the leaves, relaxation happens even before the massage begins.

When the surroundings make you feel "this is how things were meant to be," you know you've got the right place.

The right place has the right temperature. Those summer afternoons wouldn't be effective if it weren't for the sun. Temperature is an important factor to keep in mind when giving a massage. Some experts think a temperature of 70°F is adequate; I like it warmer, around 74° or 76°. The commonsense approach, of course, is to avoid either chilling or sweating. Chilled muscles contract, no matter how much you massage them. And remember, not only must the room be comfortable, but your hands must be warm, too, before you touch your friend.

Partly to prevent chilling and partly for modesty's sake, many masseurs cover the person being massaged with towels. Again, that's a matter of individual taste, upbringing and quality of relationship between those involved. In many situations, towels (or undergarments) may be appropriate.

My own preference is to give and receive massages nude when possible. My reason is simply my subjective feeling, as with my choice of environment, that "this is the way things were meant to be." It's more relaxing, refreshing, and free that way. But if being nude will create stress and tension in you or your friend, then use towels or undergarments. What's important is that you both feel comfortable. But try not to let anything come between your hands and your friend's body during the massage.

The right place has the necessary equipment. When you give a lengthy and serious massage—as opposed to a casual two-minute back rub or an erotic massage—you need to plan ahead to assure your own stamina and also that the continuity of the massage won't be interrupted. The right place is the one equipped with the essentials.

First, your stamina: Your hands are stronger than you perhaps realize. Even if you're a beginner, your hands won't wear out doing the classical massage techniques (or finger pressure either, if you follow instructions). The weak points are your back and your knees—and that's why the floor and the ground are not good places to give prolonged massage.

Yes, it's romantic to have your friend lie on the carpet in front of the fireplace or in the grass on a sunny afternoon while you give him or her a massage. But it will have to be a short massage and not as completely fulfilling as it might be, for otherwise your knees will get sore and possibly chafed, and your back will end up aching so much that *you* will be the one needing a massage. You might also get leg cramps, and the impaired circulation in your legs could cause additional discomfort.

A massage table is the first order of business. You can put one together in a matter of minutes with a solid core door and two carpenter's horses from the lumberyard. Or you can use a sturdy kitchen table, or a single or twin bed elevated on concrete blocks. If you use a bed, add a sheet of plywood above the mattress to make it firm. The surface on which your friend will lie must be firm in order to prevent sagging when you apply pressure.

The ideal table will be 30 inches from the floor if you are of average height—about level with the top of your pelvic bone. It will be about 6 feet long and 2 to 3 feet wide, giving you complete access to your friend's body from either side.

Let me stress that the table must be sturdy. I recently heard of a middle-aged man who climbed on a picnic table to have his wife massage a stiff shoulder, and received a broken wrist when the table collapsed.

Cover the table surface with a double thickness of old carpeting or carpet padding. Padding, which is about 1-inch thick foam rubber, can be purchased inexpensively by the yard at any carpet outlet. You can hold it in place on the table by draping a rubber or plastic sheet over it, then stapling the sheet securely to the underside of the table.

Finally, place a soft, absorbent cloth over the entire length of the table. Some people prefer a satin sheet, which is fine if it isn't cold against the skin. Lambskin and leather are delightful.

Once the massage begins, there should be no break in the continuity; at least one hand should always remain in contact with your friend's body. That means you should have at hand an adequate and readily available supply of the oil or lotion you're using.

Many a sad soul has drenched himself, his friend, and his living room carpet with oil in the course of a massage, so here's my recommendation for preventing that sort of thing. You'll find in your local supermarket several brands of liquid soap, each in a handy pump dispenser. Buy one, use the soap, then wash the dispenser thoroughly. When it dries, fill it with your massage oil, then tighten the lid.

The oil is instantly available with the pressing of a thumb, and if you knock the container over, it won't spill a drop.

Although most finger pressure massage doesn't require a lubri-cant, classical massage works better when one is used. The Greek physician Herodotus preferred "a greasy mixture," and today some people like fat, petroleum jelly, lanolin, cold cream, and cocoa butter. Plato and Socrates preferred olive oil. Oils are probably the most popular lubricants. Together with olive oil, neat's-foot oil and the oil of coconuts, sunflower seeds, and even corn are used. No one has proved that one is better than another, so take your choice.

My favorite lotion is a concoction of my own. To 3 ounces of olive oil I add half a teaspoon of pure oil of eucalyptus, available at any good drugstore. I like it for two reasons: It gives a slight tingling sensation to the body, and the smell reminds me of cough drops, which makes me feel as though something healthful is happening. You can get the same effect with oil of wintergreen.

And remember: about a teaspoon of oil at a time is enough.

Unless your friend asks for a small pillow, don't provide one; it will tilt the neck and shoulder muscles at an angle that will inter-fere with the massage. The exception is when support for an in-jured limb is needed, which we'll discuss later.

The Right Setting

The best massage is something of a spiritual experience, and although I'm not sure that a church would be an appropriate place, it does meet some of the basic requirements.

The right setting is one of solitude, quiet, with no fear of distur-bance

When I give massage indoors, I take the phone off the hook and ask the rest of the family not to disturb me. If my friend prefers it, I supply earplugs. Otherwise, I might play soft music on the stereo. At other times, I open the window and let the woodland sounds fill the room.

I don't talk, except to ask my friend to roll over. Your friend should be encouraged to tell you when he or she is uncomfortable. Otherwise, words interfere with the deeper communication of touch.

Bright lighting and overhead lighting are taboo. Beyond that, use lighting to set the mood you want. Sunlight beaming through a window makes a cheerful, friendly atmosphere; candlelight en-hances sensuality. For novelty, you might try a massage in total darkness. (It's like no other experience, except perhaps for the

Hawaiian practice of massaging under water.) Tensions dissolve in the darkness; your friend will forget you're there, know only your hands, and float free in pleasure.

The Right Time

I have a friend who went twice a week to a masseur, but after two months he quit the sessions because they didn't restore the relaxation and vigor he sought. The masseur was highly qualified, and the setting was tranquil. I asked him how long the massage lasted.

"A half hour," he said. "I only have an hour for lunch, and it takes me 15 minutes to get there and another 15 back."

"How can you relax when you've got to worry about getting back to the office in time?" I asked him. Today, he has an hour-long massage once each week, and it's working for him because he goes after work when there's no time clock to worry about.

The right time is when time is unimportant. There's nothing wrong with worrying or being in haste, but that's not the right time to give—or receive—a massage. The ideal is to have a whole morning or afternoon or evening free. And although you, the masseur, will not necessarily spend all that time giving a massage, it will end spontaneously, when it should, not when it must. Plan to have at least two uninterrupted hours available.

The right time is when you are prepared to devote your thoughts and feelings to your friend. When you give a massage, your hands are talking, and as long as they're touching your friend's body, you can't silence them. Your friend will hear them, either consciously or unconsciously, and he or she will respond to what they're saying. If you're distracted by worry, your hands will transfer that to your friend. If you're in haste, your friend will grow restless. It takes a highly skilled masseur, a real professional, to teach his hands to lie.

Dr. Frances M. Tappan, one of the leading authorities in physical therapy, insists in her book (*Healing Massage Techniques*) that effective massage is more than mere technique of body manipulation. "One who devotes total attention by communicating concern, empathy and sincere desire to promote the healing process will spur a patient to participate in the effort toward regaining good health."

It's important for you to be willing to let your hands speak confidently of their healing power, of your affection, of the happiness you derive from giving pleasure. That's particularly crucial when you're massaging your friend for the first time, for we of Western cultures have a peculiar sense of guilt at accepting pleasure from others when we haven't paid for it—unlike cultures of the Orient, where massage is given as a way of life, and there's no attitude of who's doing what for whom. In our society, we tend to feel that common courtesies are services that must be rewarded by tipping or payment, and when we can't do that, we feel guilty or indebted. So, if you communicate to your friend that you're receiving as much pleasure as he or she, that you're really enjoying massaging his or her body, then your friend will relax and enjoy, too.

The right time is when you're not weary but physically strong enough to give an effective massage. Fatigue is easily, if unconsciously, detected by the one you're touching, and it'll make your friend feel guilty and tense.

How long should a massage last? Every expert has his opinion, and yours is as good as theirs. Albert Hoffa, the author of *Technik der Massage,* felt 10 to 20 minutes for local massage—a specific muscle or muscle group causing pain—was ideal, whereas a general massage might last from 30 to 45 minutes. James Mennell, another important person in the field, thought that general massage should last no longer than an hour and 15 minutes. Some have described "total" massages of 30 minutes, whereas still others have insisted that a truly effective total massage must take an hour and a half.

The ancient Greek physician Galen probably offered the best advice:

> What shall be the duration of the rubbing it is impossible to declare in words; but the director (masseur) being experienced in these matters, on the first day must form a conjecture, which shall not be very accurate, but the next day, having already acquired some experience in the constitution of his subject, he will revise his conjecture continually to greater accuracy.

Your hands not only speak, they listen. As you gain experience, you'll feel the muscles of your friend's body telling you when the tension is dissipating, when the stiffness or pain has vanished, when the warm and pleasurable feeling has reached its fulfillment.

That's the right time to stop.

PART II
CLASSICAL MASSAGE FOR WHOLE-BODY RELAXATION

CHAPTER THREE

THE FUNDAMENTALS OF CLASSICAL MASSAGE

Classical massage is the caress of comfort or affection, the easing of soreness in another's body by rubbing or manipulating the pain away, the transmittal of pleasure or relaxation by firm or gentle strokes.

Massage of this sort is probably as old as the human species, originating when men and women first touched each other and their offspring, sometimes in a futile effort to restore life, sometimes to convey tenderness when words were not available, or not adequate. Massage was therapy, an experiment in kindness. It was the language of love. And it was universal.

The Greeks were the first to recognize what is now often called classical massage and to incorporate it into everyday life. No doubt, the Greeks used finger pressure techniques—just as the Chinese used what we now call classic methods—but the techniques that the Greeks emphasized (and which are a major component of massage even today) were first described by Hippocrates in 430 B.C.:

"It is necessary to rub the shoulder following reduction of a dislocated shoulder. It is necessary to rub the shoulder gently and smoothly."

The Greeks used massage for both pleasure and health. According to Homer's *Odyssey*, battle-weary warriors returned from the fields to a reward of prolonged massage administered by beautiful women. Both in public baths, which catered to lovers of pleasure, and athletic gymnasiums, which were devoted to healthy bodies, Greek males could receive elaborate massages that included pummeling, squeezing, punching, and rubbing.

The typical Greek physician studied massage, and at least one doctor, Asclepiades, devoted his practice exclusively to massage which, he believed, could cure by reestablishing the natural flow of nutritive fluids throughout the body. Only food was more necessary to life than massage, according to Socrates and Plato. The Greeks also massaged their animals.

Those who practiced classical massage claimed they could render virtually miraculous cures. Some of those claims have been proved false, but others—particularly those involving blood circulation, the muscles, and nervous system—have been substantiated.

When Rome conquered Greece, it absorbed classical massage techniques. As Roman influence spread throughout the ancient world, healers of many nations incorporated classical techniques into their own methods of massage.

All over Europe throughout the Middle Ages and Renaissance, healers continued to use massage. But until the nineteenth century it was an art rather than a science, each practitioner developing his own methods based on observation and advice from more experienced practitioners. Most masseurs had a limited repertoire of techniques, but no idea which method was best for treating a given problem.

In 1914, Peter Ling of Stockholm, Sweden, changed that, and in the process made one of the single most important contributions to massage as a science. Ling devoted many years to studying massage as practiced in Classical Greece as well as contemporary Italy, Switzerland, France, England, and Scotland. From his research he systematically organized the techniques that seemed most beneficial, and taught them at his school, the world's first institute for scientific study of massage.

The techniques Ling taught have come to be known as Swedish massage because Ling did his work in Sweden—but Western or classical massage is a more accurate term because the techniques were first described in ancient Greece.

Yet, masseurs often use French words to describe Swedish massage techniques. This is because French missionaries were the first to describe the classical-type massage techniques they found being used—in China! The French names and descriptions quickly became part of the vocabulary for masseurs throughout Europe after Ling used them.

Ling's major strokes are sliding (*effleurage*), kneading (*petrissage*), striking (*tapotement*), compression or pressure (friction), and vibration (the same in French).

Two other practitioners were widely influential. One, Albert

Hoffa, took massage a step closer to a science when he wrote the book that is still a basic text on the subject, *Technik der Massage,* in 1900. He emphasized massaging individual muscles and muscle groups, and using more pressure than was customary among some masseurs. The other was James Mennell, who had worked with patients suffering fractures and other serious injuries, and in 1917 concluded that gentle massage was preferable under all circumstances.

Most massage today, whether it's practiced in physical therapy, in a sunny field of clover, or in a Manhattan apartment, is an amalgam of techniques. Tell your neighbor you're learning to give a wonderful massage and, even though she hasn't read this book, she'll have a good idea what you mean. She might call it whole-body massage or just stroking, or if she's ever belonged to a health club, she might think of it as Swedish massage.

Who cares what you call it—it's how it's done that counts, beginning with the pattern of the strokes. That's what the following diagrams illustrate.

One aspect of classical massage that shouldn't be spontaneous is the pattern you'll follow. The strokes should form a pattern that makes it possible to give a complete massage without ever taking your hands from your friend's body. The diagrams will help you memorize the flow of the movement, using numbers which indicate "Destination Points" for reference.

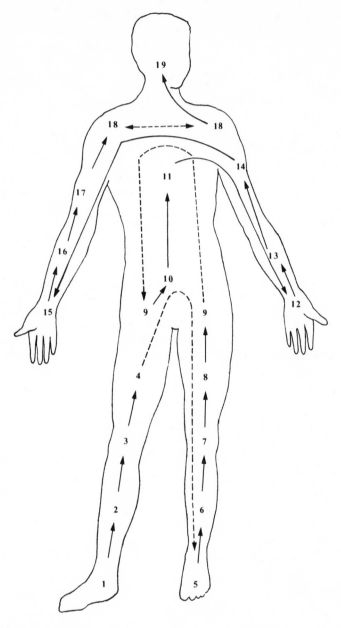

Front.

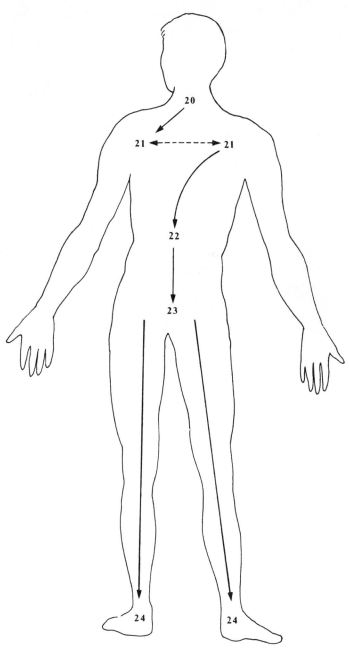

Back.

CHAPTER FOUR

STROKES AND TECHNIQUES IN CLASSICAL MASSAGE

In this chapter, you'll learn five basic strokes you'll need to master classical massage: *sliding, kneading, compression, striking,* and *vibration.* Each step of the classical massage process consists of one of these basic strokes, or a combination of several, and is designed for a specific part of the body.

Here are some points to keep in mind:

- Classical massage strokes should never cause pain. When they do, the muscle naturally contracts to protect itself, which is exactly the opposite of the result you're seeking: muscle relaxation. The amount of pressure you use depends on three factors: the stroke itself, your friend's sensitivity and preference, and the goal of the massage. In general, lighter strokes produce relaxation and a feeling of general well-being, whereas stiff muscles respond to somewhat greater pressure. But many people prefer to have their muscles really worked over, and others tense up when any significant pressure is applied. *You must always be conscious of your friend's responses and react accordingly.*
- Strokes should always be in the direction of the *venous* blood and lymph flow unless the strokes are very light. A rule of thumb: Move *from* the outer parts of the body *toward* the heart.
- Strokes should follow the direction of muscle fibers except where indicated in the text.

- Make sure your hands are clean and warm, your fingernails are short with no sharp edges, and rings, watches, and jewelry are removed.

As you learn the strokes and massage methods, remember that your own instincts should be your final guide in deciding which method, which stroke will bring pleasure or relief. This book will teach you the *skills* of massage, but developing the art is equally important.

And now—let's get started.

Sliding (effleurage)

Sliding is the fundamental stroke, the one most people know about because it's the instinctive touch we use to pet a kitten or caress a lover.

To do the sliding stroke, use your whole hand, fingers together. Your hand should fit snugly around the muscle, adapting continuously to its shape and size, so that you're always touching as much of your friend's body as possible.

There are two different types of sliding strokes. The *light sliding stroke* is used for a gentle relaxation massage, to begin every massage, as a transition between the strokes, and to conclude every massage. The *deep sliding stroke* is used for a more concentrated effect.

Light Sliding. In light sliding, the direction of the strokes isn't important, but consistency is. It's like painting a house: It doesn't particularly matter if your brush strokes are up and down or left to right as long as you stick with the pattern. The inconsistent stroke will be obvious and distracting. Also, light sliding should not be *too* light or superficial, or it will end up tickling and otherwise stimulating your friend instead of being relaxing.

Deep Sliding. Deep sliding should be done only on muscles relaxed through the superficial stroke. The technique is the same—only the amount of pressure differs. Increase the pressure by leaning into your arms—use your weight, not your muscles, and keep the pressure evenly distributed throughout your hands.

And, deep sliding strokes (like other deep strokes) should always move in the direction of the *venous* blood and lymph flow, usually from the extremities toward the heart, from the outside of the body toward the inside.

Beginners sometimes mistakenly believe they must press hard in deep sliding. That's not so. There should be no appreciable friction heat between your hands and your friend's skin, and you shouldn't feel that you're laboring at it. Keep your body—especially your back, arms, and hands—relaxed. Too much pressure will cause muscle tightness in both you and your friend.

Some people really enjoy the gentle start and finish with the subtle surge of pressure in the middle. Others enjoy the reassuring firmness of continuing pressure. There no "right" or "wrong" method, however. Allow your friend to guide you in questions like these; you'll find it much more enjoyable and effective.

Variations on Sliding

Knuckling. For more pressure on stiff or painful muscles, or on less sensitive muscles such as the back, make a fist and place the area between your knuckles and the first finger joints on the muscles you're treating. Move your hand forward, extending the fingers in a flicking motion,

Shingling. This is a superficial stroke, particularly useful for relaxation. Begin with one hand at the neck and continue gently along the spine. Before the stroke is complete, start the second stroke with the other hand a few inches below where the first one began, overlapping strokes as though you were shingling a roof.

Horizontal. This is a good deep stroke for the lower back. Place a hand at each side of your friend's back and move both with firm pressure so that they pass at the spine (don't put pressure on the spine) and cross to opposite sides. As the hands move toward each other, they'll press the muscles upward, squeezing them. As they travel apart again, they'll stretch the muscle.

(Incidentally, sliding, as with many of the other strokes, will be referred to in verb form—"to slide"—as well as in noun form.)

Kneading (petrissage)

If you can imagine yourself using one hand to squeeze empty an extra-large tube of toothpaste, you'll have some idea of the kneading stroke. To get the toothpaste out, you must wrap your hand around the bottom and squeeze the lowest part first, then the middle, finally the part beneath your thumb and first finger. Next, you must slide your hand a bit higher, overlapping the spot you just squeezed, and repeat the process until you've emptied the tube.

You can't wrap your hand around an entire muscle, but you *can* lift it—or part of it—between your thumb and fingers and squeeze it. You're not moving toothpaste but waste products in the muscle tissue, and kneading is probably the most effective stroke for doing that. Stiff and just-exercised muscles respond well to this stroke.

Relax the muscles with sliding strokes before attempting to knead, and remove excess lubricant that'll cause your friend's flesh to slip out of your grasp. Lift the muscle *gently* between thumb and fingers and milk it toward the heart. You might include an easy circular motion at the same time. Then, slide your hand to the adjoining section, closer to the heart, and repeat. Keep your hand in contact with your friend's body at all times.

You can use full-hand kneading on arm and lower leg muscles by grasping the entire muscle with the palm of your hand, lifting it and milking it.

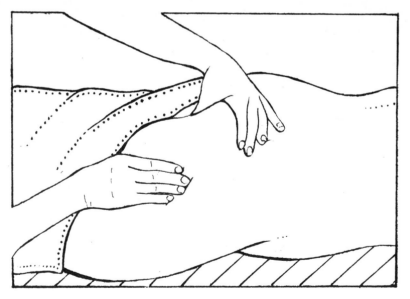

Two-hand kneading—both hands move in the same circular direction, one at the top of the circle while the other is at the bottom. The muscle is tugged first in one direction, then the other, squeezed as the hands approach, stretched as they separate.

Or, you can use two hands on large muscle groups such as those of the back and thigh. Place one hand a few inches higher than the other and keep them about 3 inches apart. Both hands move in a circular motion and in the same direction so that they pull the muscle apart, then gently pinch it together as the hands approach each other. Although the muscle isn't precisely lifted, it's pressed up, and the circular motion of the hands milk it. Slide them higher and repeat.

The keys to effective kneading:

- Go slowly. Fight the tendency to rush through it. Allow your friend to savor the sensation you're giving him or her.
- Maintain a rhythm as you move from one muscle area to the next so that the experience is a single, continuous whole, rather than a series of jerky movements.
- Go gently. Don't pinch or hurt.

Compression (friction)

This is an especially good stroke when pain, stiffness, or muscle spasm is located in a small area. It also helps loosen scar tissue and adhesions that might have built up in the muscles and connecting tissues, encourages absorption of wastes, and promotes circulation. Unlike the sliding stroke, your hands should *not* move across the skin, so lubricants can cause a problem. The goal is to cause the tissues *beneath* the skin to glide across the muscle, stimulating and warming the stiff or painful area.

Use the ball of your thumb, your fingers, or the heel of your hand to apply moderate pressure in a circular motion. Keep the movements slow and rhythmic. Remember to maintain firm contact with the skin as you stretch and loosen the underlying tissue.

Striking (tapotement)

This category includes the strokes that the silent movie era had so much fun with: pounding, clubbing, punching, and such until the subject needed hospitalization. In reality, there should be nothing remotely sadistic about these strokes, which help to stimulate muscles by causing reflex contractions and increasing the blood supply. Striking is an excellent follow-up to strenuous exercise. It's *not* recommended for painful muscles or conditions that might be exacerbated by increased muscle contraction. Striking should also not be used over the lower abdomen or lower back where sensitive organs can be bruised. Here are the major striking strokes.

Tapping. Use the fingertips. Think of your fingers as raindrops falling on your friend.

Slapping. Use your open hand or just the fingers, slap rapidly and vigorously, but not so hard that your friend tenses his body.

Cupping. The hands are partially closed so that the fingertips and the heel of the hand alone make contact.

Hacking. With palms facing each other, strike the muscles rapidly with the sides of your hands. If your hands grow tired, close them into fists (called *beating*) for a similar effect.

Vibration

This stroke is refreshing, relaxing, and stimulating to a weary body. Just rest your hands on your friend and begin a trembling motion. Unfortunately, while your friend becomes invigorated, you'll become exhausted; it's a difficult stroke to maintain for long.

Today, most masseurs use a mechanical device if they want to use the vibration stroke, and that's what I recommend. The gadget can keep on vibrating long after you collapse.

So that's all there is to it, five simple strokes: sliding, kneading, compression, striking, and vibration. With them, you can produce complete relaxation, relieve even severe muscle pain and stiffness, and promote overall health and vigor.

You should be asking me about now: "That's all well and good, but just *when* do I use *what* stroke?"

I'm glad you asked, because that's what the next chapter, "Giving a Classical Massage," is all about. You'll notice that each section flows into the next; that is, the first stroke of each section can be a continuation of the last stroke of the previous one. Keep moving, following the patterns on pages 20–21. Knowing exactly what comes next will give you a sense of confidence that you'll convey to your friend.

CHAPTER FIVE

GIVING A CLASSICAL MASSAGE

The Foot Massage

If your friend is new to massage, she might very well be embarrassed at having your hands suddenly touch her face or body. We're much less sensitive about having our feet touched. By the time you're finished with a good foot massage, your friend will be relaxed enough to enjoy what follows.

The feet "appreciate" massage perhaps more than most other parts of the body. It's not only because most feet get an enormous workout every day, but because the circulation is often poorer there, at the farthest extremity from the heart. That's why the first indication of poor circulation is usually cold, crampy feet. It's also the reason that gout-causing uric acid crystals accumulate in the joint of the big toe; circulation is insufficient to carry those crystals away as waste products. Foot massage aids the circulation, giving the feet a warm, tingling, refreshing feeling.

Besides, many of us simply enjoy having our feet played with. Maybe it reminds us of infancy; a few minutes' vacation back to the carefree contentment of childhood has to be pleasant for all of us. That's a good way to prepare your friend for all that's to come.

1. *Toe Slide.* Begin with your friend lying on his back, and you at his feet, facing them. With one hand, lift the foot by grasping it behind the heel. Place your other hand on top of the foot above the toes, conforming your hand to the shape of the foot. Slide upward

to the knee using moderate to heavy pressure. Slide back to the starting point with light pressure. (Three repetitions.)

2. Repeat the sliding stroke from toes to knee, but as one hand reaches the ankle, begin sliding with the other hand, slightly higher up the foot. (Three slow, firm repetitions.)

3. *Heel-to-Heel.* Lift your friend's foot at the ankle, and lay your other hand on the bottom of his foot, fingers against toes. Press the heel of your palm just below the ball of the foot, where the toes end, and slide down over his heel. Use heavy pressure; it will feel good. But hold the foot securely at the ankle to prevent pressure from being applied to the leg. (One or two repetitions.)

4. Make a fist and slide across the underside of the foot as you did in step 3, using the joint below your knuckles rather than the heel of your hand. Use moderate to heavy pressure. (Three repetitions.)

In massaging the bottom of the foot, the problem isn't that you'll use too much pressure usually, but too little. The foot is used to rough treatment and craves real stimulation. The same gentle touch that would bring pleasure to the face or arms will tickle the feet.

5. *Thumb Massage.* Next is a massage of the top of the foot. Grasp the foot with both hands, the heels of your thumbs on each side of the top part of the foot, your fingers on the bottom. Using the compression stroke and pressing firmly to keep the skin from slipping, rub up and down.

Holding the foot as above, move all four fingers of one hand in a circular motion on the bottom of the foot, just beneath the ball, to create a relaxing friction. Remember that in compression your fingers do not slide across the skin. Rather, the skin slides across underlying tissues. (After four repetitions, move to a lower part of the foot and repeat. Continue to the heel.)

6. *Down the Valleys.* A series of bones extend from the top of the foot to each toe, and between these toes are "valleys" where tension accumulates. Using light pressure, trace each valley individually from the top of the foot to the toe, ending with a gentle tug at the skin. (Two repetitions.)

7. *Toe Tug.* Hold the foot steady with one hand and grip the big toe at its base between your thumb and finger. Squeezing lightly, milk fresh blood forward into it. (Repeat with each toe.)

8. *Foot Tug.* Our feet are constantly being pressed toward our legs, so it can be a delightful experience to have the pressure reversed. Grasp your friend's foot with one hand at the heel and

the other just below the ankle. With firm and steady pressure, pull it toward you, but not with such force as to actually move your friend's body. Gently twist the foot to left and right. Hold for about 12 seconds, and conclude with a sliding stroke to the knee. (Three repetitions.)

The Whole-Leg Massage

To maintain unity and flow of the massage, I recommend after massaging the first foot, you continue to the leg rather than crossing to the second foot immediately. It's much more satisfying to the recipient than jumping from foot to foot or leg to leg.

In massaging legs, particularly a man's, avoid accidentally pulling out hair. The simple solution is to use enough lubricant, especially in strokes toward the heart and against the grain of hair growth.

Even if your friend is perfectly at ease, his muscles have a mind of their own; the nerves in them will respond to a sudden squeeze

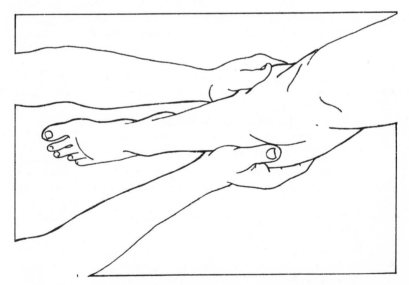

Your friend's leg must be well lubricated for the full-leg slide. Otherwise, the pressure against the grain of hair growth can be quite painful. Try adding gentle kneading when you reach major muscles.

or localized pressure by stimulating the muscle to contract. That's why the first stroke on any new body area should be light sliding. It shows your friend's involuntary nervous system that your touch is no threat and you can be trusted.

Full-leg Slide. Place a hand at each side of the ankle. Your thumbs should rest on each side of the shinbone (fibula), and your fingers should embrace the muscular underside of the leg.

Slide your hands upward, cupping the muscles so that you're actually pressing the leg muscles between thumbs and fingers. Glide gently over the knee, then resume pressure on the upper muscles (quadriceps) of the thigh.

Don't try to press with your thumbs alone. Instead, lean into the movement, using your weight to apply pressure.

Where the leg joins the torso, slide the hand on the outside part of the leg over the muscles above the hip joint, applying firm pressure. Simultaneously, bring the hand on the inside part of the lower leg to the inner thigh. Move both hands now along both sides of the leg, returning to the ankle. Unless the table is too high, this can all be done while you remain at your friend's feet.

(I hesitate to suggest a set number of repetitions of this step, because I once had a companion who found it so delightful that I spent half the night on it only, and never did get to another. The firmness of sliding up gives a sense of trust and security, and the softness of the downstroke is stimulating. In general, you should repeat this step twice, and another two times if you see that it's particularly satisfying. It might not be—we all respond differently.

The Ankle Massage

Grasp between your thumb and forefinger the flesh behind your friend's anklebone, just above the heel. Pinch it lightly for about 5 seconds, then switch to gentle circular compression. (After four repetitions, slide higher and repeat. Continue upward for about 3 inches, to the point where the tendon unites with the muscle.)

The Lower-Leg Massage

The large calf muscle (gastrocnemius) is ideal for kneading. Your hand just naturally fits around it, and kneading seems spontaneous. It's also the best way to ease the almost ticklish stiffness and ache that develops in this hard-worked muscle.

1. Start with full-hand kneading. First, place a rolled towel beneath your friend's knee (never under the ankle, which will put stress on the knee joint and make your friend contract muscles to ease the pressure). The towel will lift the lower leg from the table, so now reach behind the leg with both hands and grasp as much muscle as you can in each. The hands should be just above the ankle, one slightly higher than the other. With the lower hand, squeeze the entire muscle, letting the flesh "ooze" slowly from your grip.

As the muscles ooze out, relax the lower hand and begin squeezing with the upper one. Move the lower hand above the upper one and repeat till you reach the knee.

Return to the ankle with a light sliding stroke, thumbs on each side of the shinbone and fingers reaching around the muscle. (Three repetitions.)

2. *Calf Press.* You're going to massage from ankle to knee where the shin and muscle meet, using the compression stroke. Gently turn your friend's foot outward and bend his knee slightly so that you can work on the calf muscle. Lay three fingers in that groove just above the anklebone and use a rapid, circular motion. (One repetition, progressing slowly toward the knee.)

3. When you've reached the knee, slide the palm of your hand around the large calf muscle and, using your hand instead of your fingers, repeat step 2, this time toward the ankle. (Three repetitions.)

4. Finish with a deep sliding stroke to the knee. (Three repetitions.)

The Knee Massage

The bone known as the kneecap, or patella, is held in place by a ligament connected to the shinbone and tendons attached to the large muscles of the thigh. That constitutes little to massage in the knee itself, and in fact there's always the danger that a particularly clumsy and exuberant novice could actually cause damage to the knee in efforts to massage it.

Just above the kneecap, however, where that tendon connects to muscle, is another area that begs for massage. A combination of compression and kneading is perfect here. It'll probably be more convenient to move alongside your friend now, but continue to face his head.

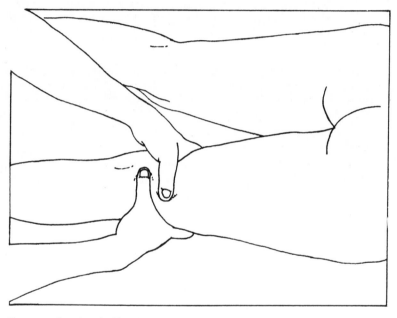

The cross-thumb rub. Thumbs move at a right angle to the leg with sufficient pressure to loosen adhesions in the area. Make sure you use enough lubricant so that your thumbs slide over the skin rather than painfully tugging at it.

1. *Cross-thumb Rub.* About an inch above the patella, you can feel on both the left and right sides the tendons as they unite with the thigh muscle. With your fingers surrounding the leg, put your thumbs on these tendons. Rub *across* rather than parallel to the tendons so that you can feel them rippling beneath your thumbs. Use enough pressure to keep the skin from slipping (compression), and bring your thumbs toward each other, then away (kneading). (Five slow repetitions.)

2. *Palm Compression.* Place your open hands on the sides of the thigh, the heels of your hands just above the knee bone. Press firmly and move your hands in a circular motion. Don't let your hands move against the skin surface, but make the inner tissues slide against each other and build friction. (Three repetitions.)

The Thigh Massage

The large muscle groups of the thigh, like those of the buttocks, forearms, and shoulders, "appreciate" just about every stroke, and you should feel free to use your own creativity and imagination, as well as sensitivity to your friend's responses.

1. *Long Slide.* Always start by sliding with moderate pressure from the knee along the top of the thigh to the hip and groin, then along the sides of the leg and back to the knee. The return motion should always be light. It can be done with just the fingers, whereas for the upward motion you should use your entire hand contoured to the shape of the muscle. (Three repetitions.)

2. *Whole-hand Knead.* Stand beside your friend's thigh, facing it. Grasp the muscle with both hands just above the knee. Your thumbs should be on the outer side of the thigh, your palms on the top, and your fingers on the inner thigh, pointing down. Squeeze the muscle up into the palms of both hands. While tugging the muscle toward your friend's hip with your upper hand, pull the lower hand outward (toward you). Slide a bit higher along the leg and repeat, continuing until you are just below the hip.

By turning the foot outward and flexing the knee as you did for the calf, you can reach the large flexors, the muscles at the back of the thigh. Repeat the same kneading motion that you used on the front of the thigh. (Three repetitions.)

3. *Transition Strokes.* End with short shingling strokes from the knee to the hip and across the abdomen. Use long, light sliding strokes down the opposite leg to the foot. Repeat the entire process, beginning with step 1 of the foot massage.

Abdomen and Chest

I can't conceive of giving a *total* massage without spending a good deal of time and attention on the chest and abdomen. There are many reasons, both psychological and physical:

- Circulation of all the lower extremities, both superficial and deep, can be enhanced through abdominal massage. (Some experts claim that abdominal massage can thereby dramatically affect sexual performance and pleasure. I've seen no proof of that—yet, the logic appears sound. Improved circulation would, it seems, have some beneficial effect.)
- Neck and back pain can often be relieved through chest and abdominal massage. No mystery here. The pectoralis major— the chest muscle that makes weight lifters look like they should be wearing bras—attaches to bone structures that affect the alignment of the upper body. Tightness in the pectoralis can produce any number of structural compensations and abnormal stresses. The same is true of lower abdominal muscles and back pain.

The Whole-Body Massage

Remember the pump-type oil dispenser mentioned earlier? Here's where it becomes important. If you try to massage a hairy body without lubricant, you'll hear screeches—and they won't be screeches of pleasure. So be sure to lubricate your hands, without breaking complete contact with your friend, as you do the following *transition strokes.*

1. As you finish the final upward shingling stroke of the second leg, continue with the outer hand over the hip and waist, along the rib cage toward the armpit. The inner hand crosses the lower abdomen just above the pubic bone to the other hip and upward along the far side of the body. Both hands should arrive at the pectoral muscles of the chest below the clavicle simultaneously. This is a superficial motion with open hands that shape to the contours of your friend's body. (Three repetitions.)

2. Bring your hands together, with your thumbs over the sternum, or breastbone. Slide them down the center of your friend's body. Use very light pressure over the bone, increasing to moderate pressure beneath the ribs. Your fingers should be flat and pointing toward your friend's head. (Three repetitions.)

3. When the heels of your hands reach the pubic bone, slide your fingers outward and continue around the waist. Your hands are now at your friend's sides. Slide them upward to your friend's armpits again. (Repeat two more times.)

The Abdomen Massage

Although professionally trained practitioners occasionally use heavy pressure on the abdomen, the potential dangers are too great for the layperson to risk. Direct your massage at the *muscles* of the abdomen rather than the *organs* beneath them. The fact is, stimulation of the nerves and blood supply of the muscles *will* affect the organs beneath.

1. ***Triangular Slide.*** As you finish the whole-body strokes, still standing at your friend's side, your hands will come to rest above the pubic bone. Turn your fingers outward and slide to the waist, as though repeating step 3 of the whole-body massage. Now, grasp the waist securely and press the heels of your hands toward each other gently—a compression stroke. Next, slide your hands together toward the center of your friend's body, your fingers tracing the rib cage. When your thumbs meet at the center of your friend's abdomen, bring your hands straight down to the pubic bone. (Four repetitions.)

2. ***Reverse Triangular Slide.*** Repeat step 1 in reverse—with two exceptions. Move at about half the speed and pause beneath the navel to provide a few seconds of moderate pressure. The triangle this time is from pubic bone to sternum, then down and out to the waist, where you press before returning to the pubic bone. (Three repetitions.)

3. ***Belly Knead.*** Stand at your friend's side, facing her hips. Grasp with both hands the flesh of her abdomen at the side nearest you, one hand at the level of her navel, the other lower. Squeeze the skin and tissue gently between your thumbs and fingers. Lift it, pinching or tugging. Slide an inch forward—across the abdomen —and repeat. Continue to the far side. Return with a light sliding stroke, fingers together and thumbs extended. (Three repetitions.)

4. ***Friction Circle.*** Steps 4 through 7 dramatically increase abdominal circulation. You'll see the reddening, and it feels good to your partner.

Start with the palm of one hand on the lower abdomen, the heel of your hand just above the pubic bone. Using moderate but firm pressure, move your hand in a circular motion large enough to involve the whole abdomen. This is a compression stroke, not a sliding stroke. (Eight repetitions.)

5. Now slide the fingers of both hands deeply along the hip-bone, followed by firm, circular compression strokes. The left hand should go clockwise, the right counterclockwise. (Four slow repetitions.)

6. Slide up the sides of your friend's body to the rib cage and repeat the circular compression stroke as described above. (Three slow repetitions.)

7. Use the sliding stroke slowly, with moderate pressure along the center of the body to the pubic bone. (Repeat the entire circle once.)

The Chest Massage

After completing the friction circle do a whole-torso sliding motion as the transition to the chest area. Transitions in massage are as important as they are in music and literature—without them, the most perfectly executed parts don't fit together as a whole. It's best to complete one whole-torso slide, from hips to armpits to chest and back to the pubic bone, then return along the sides to the armpits to begin the chest strokes.

The next two steps are easiest done if, without lifting your hands from your friend's body, or distracting him, you can move behind him so that you're bending over his head.

1. *Pectoral Kneading.* Continue sliding up to the chest, along the outer edge of the pectorals to the clavicle and inward to the sternum. Use light pressure with an open hand. (Continue this circling pattern lightly for three repetitions, your hands covering the entire pectoral surface.)

On the last repetition, stop at the outer edge of the pectorals at the armpit. Grasp this muscle in the palm of your hand, fingers beneath and heel above, and knead. Use firm but not painful pressure, allowing the muscle to slip slowly out of your grasp. Slide your hand an inch lower along the muscle and repeat.

If your friend is male, continue kneading to the nipples, but use light pressure there. If your friend is female, use kneading only to the breasts, then use a three-finger sliding stroke beneath them to the sternum, upward and outward to the sides. Here, use light, open palm motions, moderate pressure forward, light pressure back. (Two repetitions.)

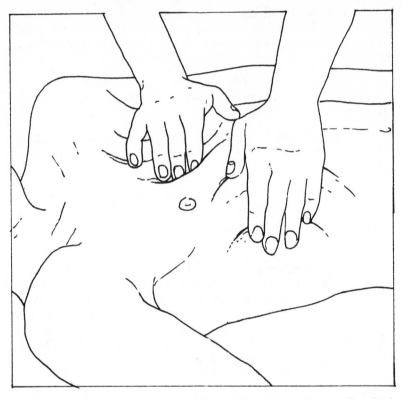

The rib press—after firmly pressing the ribs together, slide gently across the chest, hands moving in opposite directions.

2. **Rib Press.** Massage of the rib cage itself offers little benefit either physically or psychologically. The muscles are difficult to reach, and too much pressure there pinches skin and nerves against bone, a less than enjoyable experience. What's more, you can't stimulate circulation of blood or lymph by lightly massaging the rib cage.

The rib press, however, can affect lymph circulation while giving your friend a secure and cared-for feeling. Stand at her side, facing her ribs, the hand closest to her feet reaching across to her far side. Your upper hand should be in the same position on her near side. Slowly exert pressure to push the ribs together. Hold the pressure for a few seconds, then slide your hands toward each other. (Two repetitions.)

Obviously, the pressure shouldn't be so great as to fracture bones or cause discomfort. Rather, it should be like an embrace.

End this step by bringing your two hands to the center of your friend's body and sliding upward across the breasts, then to the shoulder nearest you.

Hands and Arms

Our hands and arms are almost always in action. We lift them over our heads, wave them, carry with them, push, tug—and massage. So, we rarely hear of circulatory problems in the arms and hands. That constant motion helps to pump the blood back to the heart, and keep it from pooling.

That's good. But there's a negative aspect to all that motion, too, especially when the activity is limited day after day and year after year to a certain set of motions. Too many of us know the fiery pain of a muscle torn by sudden movement because it has grown too short from lack of use. We've dismissed inflamed joints as "normal" arthritis, when actually they're the result of our failing to articulate—or use—the joints through their full range of motion. Waste products collect in such areas and eventually can cause total immobility of the joint.

As every athlete knows, muscles that work hard get stiff, short, and inflexible, unless the athlete also does stretching exercises. The problem isn't that the muscles are used, but that the use is selective. One set of muscles is overworked, whereas the opposing ones are ignored. Joints are worked in one direction and not in others.

Hand and shoulder massage, done regularly, can help to prevent or retard some of these problems. But a word of caution: If your friend is already suffering severe arthritis, get a doctor's approval before massaging the area. Never massage an inflamed or painful area; it can cause bone or tissue damage or spread an infection.

Hand Massage

1. *Transition Strokes.* The chest massage ended at the shoulder. Proceed to bring both of your hands around the shoulder to the biceps, the upper arm muscle that body builders enjoy showing

off. Using light pressure, slide one hand toward the elbow. Before this hand reaches the elbow, begin sliding the other hand along the arm as well. Continue with a light shingling stroke to the hand. (Three repetitions.)

2. *Thumb Heel Rub.* As you finish step 1, lift your friend's palm up in both of yours. Each of your thumbs should be at the base of each of the fleshy surfaces on the upper part of his hand. The obvious one (the *thenar eminence*) begins at the base of your friend's thumb, and the other (the *hypothenar eminence*) begins about an inch above the base of the little finger. Together they form the heel of the hand. Using rather heavy pressure, apply alternating pressure with one thumb then the other toward the wrist. Use light pressure when moving the thumbs back away from the wrist. (Four repetitions.)

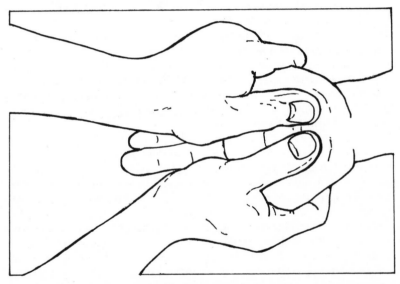

The thumb heel rub is particularly pleasurable for people who work with their hands. Use your fingers to pull the hand firmly open and your thumbs to apply alternating pressure at the base of the fleshy surfaces.

3. *Finger-Palm Slide.* Grasp your friend's thumb between your middle finger and your own thumb so that the balls of the thumbs touch. Squeeze firmly, as though forcing the blood out of the finger. Relax and move wristward to repeat the squeeze. Continue

to the top of the joint near the wrist. Squeeze the joint at the center of the wrist, then along the thumb down to the tip. Use as much pressure as you can without causing discomfort. (After two repetitions, proceed to the next finger, and so on.)

4. *Hand Stretch.* Hold your friend's palm downward in both your hands, your fingers pressing into his palm, the heels of your hands together at the back of his hand. Press firmly upward with your fingers, down and outward with your palms, as though cracking his hand in half (but don't do it). Let your hands slide sideways, gradually easing the pressure. (Two repetitions.)

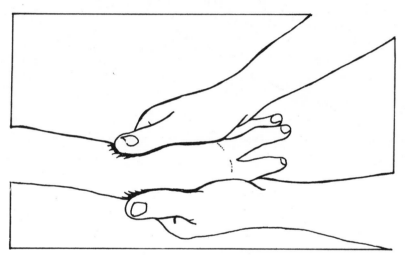

The hand stretch is surprisingly effective in relieving stiffness in the hand's many muscles and joints. Press into the palm with your fingers, outward and downward with your thumbs.

Lower-Arm Massage

The muscles of the lower arm, or forearm, give the hand its strength. Squeeze your fist, and you can see those muscles bulge. They're strong and sometimes tight, but they're great fun to massage because they're just the right size to wrap your hand around. The bones don't interfere with your ability to work the muscles, as they do in the ribs and feet. And if you want to give a deep massage, you can do it without causing pain.

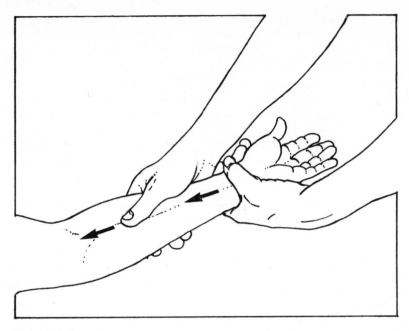

Thumb press.

1. *Transition Strokes.* Begin with a few whole-arm sliding strokes, wrist to shoulder, and return. Use one hand, shaping it to the entire muscle, or two—one above the other. (Three repetitions.)

2. *Thumb Press.* Rest your friend's arm palm up on the table, the elbow slightly bent, and grasp her wrist with your inner hand— the hand closest to her body. Lay the thumb of your other hand along her arm, pointing toward her elbow, your fingers on the underside of her arm. Press moderately with a sliding stroke along the center of the arm toward the elbow.

As you proceed, tighten the grip of your fingers. Conclude the step by squeezing out the muscle below the elbow. (Two repetitions.)

Switch hands, holding with the outer one and pressing with the thumb of the inner. (Two repetitions.)

3. *Forearm Knead.* Place the fingers of both hands around the pinkie side of your friend's arm near the wrist, your thumbs around the thumb side, and knead with moderately heavy pres-

sure. Use shingling to continue the movement to the shoulder and armpit. (One repetition.)

The Upper-Arm Massage

The upper arm is divided into three major muscle groups: the deltoid, or shoulder muscle, which actually extends almost half-way along the outer part of the upper arm toward the elbow; the triceps, on the back of your arm, which tightens when you sit at a table, put your fist on it, and press downward; the biceps, which bulge when you bend your elbow and clench your fist. It's impor-tant that you learn to identify these muscles in your own body, because you'll want to massage them separately for your friend.

Before beginning work on these specific muscle groups, you might want to give another whole-arm stroke, ending it just above the elbow, where you can begin the following.

1. *Triceps Knead.* Bend your friend's elbow outward slightly so that you can reach the triceps with your outer hand. While sup-porting the arm at the elbow with your inner hand, grasp the muscle between the thumb and index finger of your outer hand and squeeze moderately. Move farther up the arm and repeat. Continue until you reach the armpit.

If the muscle seems particularly tight and you want to spend more time on it, move to the far side of your friend without break-ing contact, lean over him and, wrapping the fingers of both hands beneath the muscle, gently pinch the flesh with both of your thumbs. Remember, it's not pressure but patience that helps the muscle to relax—too much pressure will make muscles contract and spasm.

Continue to the deltoid and return with sliding strokes to the elbow joint. (Two repetitions.)

2. *Biceps Knead.* This step is the same as the triceps knead except that the inner hand does the kneading while the outer gives support beneath the elbow. (Three repetitions.)

3. *Deltoid Slide and Knead.* Usually, you can use rather heavy pressure on the powerful deltoid muscle without causing pain. Most people find pressure soothing here, but for some it's uncom-fortable, so try to be sensitive to your friend's reaction and adapt accordingly.

Rest your friend's arm on the table, palm down. The sliding part of the deltoid slide and knead begins with your thumbs on each side of his arm and parallel to it, at the point where you feel the muscle begin.

Alternately move one hand slowly up to the shoulder bone (but don't put pressure on the bone itself), then lightly down while the other hand starts upward. Most of the pressure should be exerted by the thumbs. (Five repetitions.)

In kneading the deltoid, each hand covers the same surface as it did while sliding, except that only one hand works at a time, and the thumb and fingers squeeze the muscle rather than sliding over it: a combination of kneading and shingling.

If you find that pressure in a certain part of the muscle gives pleasure, concentrate on that area with both hands. Without breaking contact, move to the far side of the table, lean over your friend, and use the thumbs and fingers of both hands to knead the muscle.

Women usually have smaller deltoid muscles then men do. If your friend is a woman and if your hands are large and strong enough, you might try kneading the entire deltoid muscle with one hand. (Two repetitions.)

4. *Transition Strokes.* Finish the arm massage with one more light whole-arm slide. Then, proceed across the chest to massage the other arm, ending at the shoulder.

Head, Face, and Neck

A 22-year-old man told me some months ago that, because of the pressures of his job, marriage, and newly achieved fatherhood, it was simply impossible for him to relax. I saw the tension in his face, in the tapping fingers and bouncing foot as he sat in the living room, chain-smoking.

He asked me to give him a back massage. To my surprise, even that didn't entirely relax him at first. Then, I began massaging his head and face.

In the next few minutes his body visibly relaxed. His eyes closed and he breathed rhythmically in long, deep breaths. For the first time in many months he felt complete relaxation.

Many people consider the head and face so intimate a part of their bodies that they'll become tense rather than relaxed if you initiate a massage at their heads. Yet, if you establish *faith prestige,* or trust based on the ability you've demonstrated, you can move from the previous strokes to your friend's head without disturbing the serenity you've brought about. Then you can do something that I can't explain, although I've seen and experienced it many times: You can help your friend relax so thoroughly that in some cases it becomes almost a trancelike state. And, according to physical therapists who treat hospital patients, head and face massage is an excellent sedative, inducing sleep.

The Head Massage

1. *Transition Strokes.* Begin by bringing both hands across the shoulders to the neck, sliding one hand lightly up and down the front of the throat twice, thumb on one side, fingers on the other. On the third sliding stroke, use both hands, one on each side of the neck, thumbs on top, fingers together pointing to the ears. Continue to the temples. (No repetitions.)

2. *Scalp Knead.* You're still standing beside your friend, facing his head. With your fingers at his temples, make six very slow, circling movements with your fingers, using sliding rather than compression. (Such a seemingly insignificant factor as the sound of his hair brushing against your fingers actually enhances the relaxation effect. But remember: In scalp massage, never slide firmly against the grain of the hair—that can cause considerable pain to your friend.)

Slide your hand higher until your palms rest at the temples and your open fingers grasp most of the scalp. Now, squeeze rhythmically for at least 30 seconds, as though kneading dough. Remember to press your palms together against the temples each time your fingers squeeze. (Three repetitions.)

3. *Knuckle Vibe.* While keeping your fingers against your friend's head, lift your palms and slide them over your friend's ears. Very lightly, move your hand in slow circles over the ears. This is a transition step, uniting the good feelings of the scalp with the rest of the face.

Your hands still on the ears, curl your fingers in to form a fist. The part of your fingers between the knuckles and lower joints now rests against the sides of the head. Begin a trembling, or vibrating, movement that tugs the ears toward the top of the head. Press firmly enough to make the skin of the scalp move over the bones (compression). Continue for about 30 seconds, moving gradually to the center of the head and forward so that when you finish your palms are at the sides of your friend's forehead. (Three repetitions.)

4. **Deep Scalp Massage.** It's been claimed that frequent and vigorous scalp massage can stimulate new hair growth in people who are growing bald. I don't know of any scientific studies that support the idea, but I *do* know that massage will stimulate the blood supply to the skin, open clogged pores, and do more for overall scalp health than anything else I can think of, including a good shampoo.

There's nothing fancy about a deep scalp massage. You can do any or all of three things: With open hands and fingers spread, knead every part of the scalp, starting at the forehead, working back over the ears, around the base to the neck, then straight up the middle and back to the forehead; follow the same pattern with open hands, fingers together and relying on the palms to use compression, making four circles before moving to the next area; use your closed fist, knuckles down, for the vibration stroke. (Three repetitions.)

A thorough scalp massage is time-consuming and strenuous, so I don't recommend that you include it as part of a general massage until you've built strength and endurance. But when you have only 15 or 20 minutes to spend on a mini-massage, you could do a lot worse than to devote that time to your friend's head.

If you're going to use vibration on the scalp for an extended time, consider a mechanical vibrator—as most professionals do. It's one of those rare instances in massage when a machine can be more effective than you can. (See Chapter Twelve, "Mechanical Equipment.")

The Face Massage

1. **Forehead Stretch.** Slide your hands down from the scalp until your thumbs are side by side in the center of your friend's forehead and the heels of your hands are resting over her eyes. Your fingers still rest on the scalp. They act as a pivot, or anchor, as your hands slide outward toward your friend's temples in a slow, soothing motion.

When you reach the temples, move the palms in two or three firm circles.

While fingers maintain contact, lift the palms and return to the center of the forehead. (Three repetitions.)

2. *The Cheek Stretch.* Slide your hands downward so that your fingertips rest on the forehead, your hands encompass your friend's cheeks, and your thumbs rest lightly on either side of her nose. Your fingers should be turned inward toward each other so that the index fingers touch at their tips. Think of them as anchored there, acting as pivots, as you slide the palms of your hands outward with moderate pressure across the cheeks. (Four repetitions.)

This is a simple stroke, but perhaps the most basic in facial massage because it has at least three benefits. First, like the temple and forehead strokes, it relaxes. Second, it affects the major face muscles, with the same benefits that massage brings to any muscle group. In Chapter Six you'll learn how to give a facial massage specifically to enhance beauty and restore a youthful complexion, but you'll notice even now, with this step alone, that the skin becomes flushed as oxygen-rich blood comes closer to the surface beneath your hands.

Finally, the movement of your hands causes a mechanical reac-

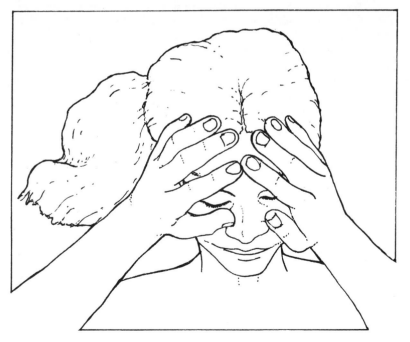

The cheek stretch involves friction. Don't slide across the skin, but tug it gently, stretching facial muscles with light pressure.

tion, as muscles are gently pressed in uncommon directions. That sets up a tugging against nasal structures that can help to open clogged sinuses and improve breathing.

3. **Nose Rub.** Return to the starting point of the last step, your thumbs on either side of the nose. Now, slide them down the nose with medium to firm pressure to the point where the cheekbone begins. Keep your thumbs away from the nostrils—your friend will find it difficult to relax if she thinks you're suffocating her.

While your thumbs move downward, allow your fingers to slide outward to the temples. Anchor them there so they can act as a pivot.

Press your thumbs firmly for several seconds in that space where the cheekbone starts away from the nose. You might want to add a very short circular or sliding motion to loosen congestion, but limit the movement to half an inch in each direction.

Now, move one thumb up along the nose toward the eye socket, then back down. As that thumb descends, the other begins to move upward in a combination of kneading and sliding. (Three repetitions.)

4. **Eyebrow Press.** First, make sure that if your friend wears contact lenses, they've been removed prior to massage. Otherwise, skip steps 4 and 5.

Conclude the last step with both thumbs at the top of your friend's nose next to the eyes. Move your thumbs up and out along the underside of the eyebrow bone. With moderate pressure, trace this bone outward, putting very light pressure on your friend's eyelids as your thumb brushes across them.

Lift your thumbs and return to the base of the nose, while pressing firmly with your fingers against your friend's temples to assure her you haven't broken contact. (Four repetitions.)

5. Bring your thumbs to the inner edge of the eyebrow and slide outward with firm pressure. (Note this: In step 4 you moved in *under* the bone; in this step, your thumb is definitely *on* the bone's outer edge and *away* from the eye.)

With your fingers still anchored at the temples, place your thumbs at the bridge of the nose next to the eyes. Move your thumbs outward across the eyelids very slowly and with minimal pressure. This will make your friend feel reassured, relaxed, and probably sleepy. (Three repetitions.)

The Neck Massage

Of the several muscles in the neck, the major one, the trapezius, is also among the largest muscles of the body. The trapezius begins about halfway down your back and connects to your spine all the way up to your skull. The muscle forms a V-shape across your back, and continues over the upper part of your shoulder. If you feel that muscle on your upper back, you'll notice that the trapezius also extends along your neck to the base of your skull.

We suffer neck pain and muscle tension in the trapezius, and there's no mystery as to why the tension hits us here. Every animal has a way of reacting to the threat of danger. A cat arches its back. A dog puts its ears back. A peacock spreads its tail. And humans bring their shoulders up and forward.

That response probably prepared us for physical combat in our cave-dwelling days, and today it remains as natural a physiological response to danger as our increased heart and breathing rate, stepped-up adrenaline excretion, and thickening of blood. These are wonderful preparations for going out to slay a tyrannosaur, and if we did face such strenuous physical exercise, it would dissipate the physiological responses to stress that accumulate destructively.

Unfortunately, few of our stresses can be dealt with physically. You might *want* to punch the boss, but you need the job. Breaking a dish over your husband's head might help to relieve the tension in the trapezius muscles, but it won't do much for your marriage. The result is that we tense up and, because we remain sedentary, we never get rid of that tension.

Pinch those trapezius muscles in your own body or your friend's and chances are they'll be hard as a rock. Squeeze the neck muscles where they spread out toward the shoulder. Lay the palm of your hand on that part of the shoulder and press your fingers into your back. Press your fingers into the back of your neck. Feel the tightness in all those areas.

If your friend is one of the many who have chronic tension of the trapezius, these muscles might never completely relax, even during sleep, without your intervention. Here's what you can do.

1. *Shoulder Squeeze.* Standing at your friend's side, press the palms of both hands on the upper shoulder muscle, your thumbs alongside the neck, your fingers around the back. Knead gently, squeezing with the heels of your hands and fingers. (Repeat at

least 10 times or until you feel some relaxation, then gradually increase the pressure until you're massaging deeply.)

You must be particularly sensitive to the response of your partner. If the pressure is too great, some people will protectively tense these muscles. Others won't begin to relax until the pressure is increased.

2. *Neck Press.* Steps 2 through 4 are done while you stand behind your friend's head. Maintain contact while moving to the new position by first gliding the hand *opposite* the side on which you're standing along his neck to the temple. (If you're on his left side, use your right hand.) When your hand reaches his temple, move around to his head, simultaneously bringing your hand slowly onto his throat and to the other temple. Take your time, think about what you're doing, and chances are your friend won't even know you've moved.

With one hand, gently lift your friend's head at the base of his skull. With the other hand grasp the back of his neck just above the shoulders and squeeze gently, increasing to moderate pressure. Slide about an inch toward the skull and repeat.

At the base of the skull, find the indentation above the last vertebra. Without pulling the hair, move one or two fingers in a circular compression stroke. (Five repetitions.)

3. *Neck Stretch.* With one hand beneath the chin and the other at the base of the skull, apply gradual and even pressure with both hands to stretch the neck. More than moderate pressure might cause the muscles to contract defensively. (Three repetitions.)

4. *The Coup de Grace.* If your friend is ever going to relax totally, he'll do it now. Gently lay his head back on the table. Massage his temples in circular sliding strokes for at least 20 seconds. Then, anchoring your fingers there, bring your thumbs parallel in the middle of his forehead. Lightly, using the entire thumbs, move outward. (At least eight repetitions.)

Now, lightly brush the hands over the ears toward the scalp. (Four repetitions.)

Cup each ear in the palm of your hand and press with moderate force. Make no movement, just hold the pressure firm for at least one minute. This is a good time to study your friend's face. You'll see neither smile nor frown, but a total sleeplike absence of tension. You can't imagine the peace he feels until you've tried it yourself.

Very gradually ease the pressure. Bring your hands down to the table and away. (Three repetitions.)

Wait patiently until your friend "returns." It might be just a few seconds—or, if he's fallen asleep, it could be much longer. There's no law that says the massage can't end right here, with his sleeping. Only when he opens his eyes should you ask him to roll over.

The Back

If my repeated instructions so far to use light, gentle pressure have been somewhat frustrating to you, and you really can't wait to get your hands into your friend's muscles in earnest, this section will make you happy. The large, sweeping back muscles, along with those of the buttocks, delight in firm treatment—it's no myth that the geisha of Japan walk barefoot on the backs of their clients as part of the completely satisfying massages they give. When I receive massage, I prefer my back to be treated almost roughly; on the other hand, my wife, although enjoying heavy pressure on her back, prefers a more gentle technique. Once again: You are the final expert on what pleases your friend.

This caution, however: Heavy pressure should never be applied to the spine or other bony areas. That pinches nerves between your hands and the bones—and it hurts. What's more, it's not impossible to push the vertebrae out of alignment, causing serious problems.

The Whole-Back Massage

As always, the first step is an "introduction" to the area you'll be massaging next.

1. *Transition Strokes.* You're still standing at your friend's head. Slide one hand lightly along the neck and the spine to the buttocks. Repeat this motion with your other hand before the first is finished, then again with the first (shingling). While one hand remains in contact with your friend's back, fill the other with a teaspoon of oil and apply it to the entire surface.

Place the heel of each hand on each side of the spine, your fingers together, pointing to the sides. Your thumbs should be parallel to the spine. Lean forward so that your weight presses the palms and heels of your hands down firmly, and slide slowly toward the buttocks. Squeeze lightly with the flat part of your fingers.

At the hips, ease pressure and slide your hands outward to the sides, then toward you, fingers pointing to the hips. Before you reach the armpits (some people are ticklish there, remember), sweep your hands back to the starting position. (Three repetitions.)

There are three more steps in whole-back massage that are very effective. You can do them all at once as introductory steps or, as I prefer, intersperse them between massaging the various muscle groups—like a recurrent and unifying theme in music.

2. **Cross-Kneading.** First is cross-kneading. Move to your friend's side and reach across his back near his armpit with one hand. Press your other hand against his near side, an inch or two lower. Simultaneously and with heavy pressure press the hands toward each other so that they'll pass at the spine and continue on to opposite sides. Go lightly over the spine.

This movement pushes muscles together, then stretches them, loosening adhesions and freeing wastes trapped between tight cells. Don't be afraid to use force—the average person could use almost all his strength without causing discomfort.

Slide your hands a little lower, overlapping the area previously covered, and repeat until you reach the *sacrum,* the large bony surface where the spine ends. (Three repetitions.)

3. **Push and Pull.** Standing at your friend's head, put your hands on her back near her neck, with your fingers pointing toward each other. On either side of the spine you'll feel a groove, and your fingers should rest in it.

Press firmly, using your weight, in a downward motion toward her buttocks. Move slowly and put no pressure on the spine. When your hands reach the sacrum, move them outward to the waist.

As your hands reach your friend's sides, your fingers should point toward her toes. Now, keeping your fingers open, press your hands toward each other and pull back toward the armpits. As you pull steadily, in a very slow slide up your friend's sides, she'll feel as though her body is growing lighter, that you're stretching her. (Two repetitions are sufficient.)

4. **The Back Hack.** Hacking and other striking strokes often relieve muscle tension when other methods fail. I can't offer research to explain why, but my theory is this: A muscle tenses or spasms because some "insult"—the medical term for external injury or abuse—signals the brain to tighten the muscle protec-

tively. When the muscle is hacked *gently* and continuously, the brain eventually recognizes this stream of insults as harmless—not much different, I suppose, than a wild animal who after frequent association with humans, begins to ignore them. The brain lumps the original insult with the hacking, ignores both, and relaxes.

Hacking should be done over the major muscles of the back, particularly where stiffness or pain exist, but *not* over bones and *not* forcefully. Also, it's a good idea to avoid the kidneys, which are located below the last rib you feel in the back.

Use the sides of your hands, beginning below the shoulder blade and slicing rapidly but not forcefully along the back. You can continue across the buttocks if you wish, then up the opposite side to the shoulder blade. Go slow—the entire step should take at least a minute. (Three repetitions.)

The Trapezius Massage

You're already familiar with the first of the two major back muscles, the trapezius, which covers not only the upper shoulder and neck but extends completely across your upper back, from shoulder to shoulder, then forms a sharp V to approximately the center of your back. The trapezius plays a major role in keeping your face from falling smack onto the typewriter keys—it's always holding our heads back against the pull of gravity unless   e're sitting or standing upright, or lying down.

1. *The Shoulder Pinch.* Standing behind your friend, grasp the tight muscle from the neck to the shoulder between your thumbs and fingers. Squeeze and knead gently because this is usually a sensitive and painful area. Move very slowly from the neck to the shoulders and back. (Two repetitions.)

This muscle sometimes responds more readily to light striking. Use the tips of your fingers only, covering the whole area. (Three repetitions.)

2. *Upper-Back Knuckling.* Fold your fingers back to the heels of your hands so that the lower half of your fingers is flat. Place those surfaces on the muscles you've just massaged, about halfway between the neck and shoulders, and press firmly, moving to the back and in toward the spine. Don't use the pointy knuckles but the flat fingers. Continue moving closer to the spine until you

reach the midpoint of the back. (You might actually be able to feel the shape of the muscle if your friend's body is well-developed.)

Return to the starting point with a light sliding stroke allowing your fingers to open. Repeat, beginning closer to the neck. (Two or three repetitions.)

3. *Two-hand Kneading.* This step begins at the outer edge of the back just above the armpit and continues to the midback near the spine.

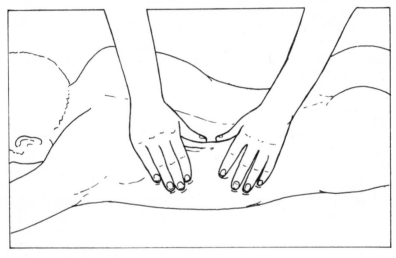

Two-hand kneading.

Standing at your friend's side, reach across him and put one hand on the lower edge of the far shoulder blade and your other hand a few inches below it and to the outside. Extend your thumbs so that they touch. Press your fingers up toward your thumbs and the thumbs down toward the fingers, squeezing your friend's back muscles between them. Continue kneading across the back to the sacrum, then slide to the starting point and repeat, this time ending higher on the spine. (When you're finished, move to your friend's opposite side without breaking contact and repeat the entire step.)

The Latissimus Dorsi Massage

This is the largest muscle of the back. It extends from the armpit to the lower back, and it's the muscle responsible for most lower back pain. In fact, some experts estimate that 80 percent of lower back pain results because this muscle isn't stretched enough. It becomes short and tight. Then, any sudden strain tears it and causes it to spasm.

Here's a bonus you didn't pay for, a jiffy course in preventing or treating lower back pain of muscular origin. Sit on the floor with your legs stretched out in front of you, feet together and knees straight. Bend forward, dropping your chin to your chest, to see how close you can come to touching your forehead to your knees. If you make virtually no progress, you're a prime candidate for lower back pain—perhaps you already suffer from it.

In attempting the exercise, you'll feel pain in your hamstrings (the muscles at the back of your thighs) and in the latissimus dorsi. The solution is to stretch and loosen those muscles. At least once a day, sit on the floor and try to touch your head to your knees. You won't be able to do it at first, and you certainly shouldn't force it. Just get as close as you can without causing real pain. Don't bob up and down, just hold that position. Remarkably, after 20 or 30 seconds, you'll feel the muscles relax and the pain subside. Then, lower yourself a bit more. Within a couple of weeks, your head will touch your knees and you won't have to worry about muscle pain in the lower back from shortened muscles.

Even those already suffering from back pain have been helped by this exercise. The pain will be much greater at first and you must proceed more gingerly, but you can actually "persuade" a muscle in spasm to relax through this steady stretching pressure. Finger pressure massage (discussed in Part III), combined with stretch exercises, can work virtual miracles in relieving back pain. (For additional stretch exercises, see Chapter 14.)

Remember, you must tuck your head in and *curl* forward to stretch the muscles of the lower back.

1. *Heel Slide.* Standing at your friend's side, place one open hand on her lower back, the heel near the far side of her spine, your thumb extended parallel to it, and your fingers together and at a right angle to the spine. Lay your other hand on top of the first and, with heavy pressure, slide your hands outward to your friend's side. Return with a lighter stroke and repeat, overlapping

the first stroke as you shingle upward on the back. (When you reach the shoulder blade, move to your friend's opposite side and repeat the entire series.)

2. **Forearm Rub.** Here's a stroke reserved for the tough muscles that need real pressure. It's ordinary sliding, but it's done with the forearm in order to cover a larger surface and apply firmer pressure than is possible with your hands.

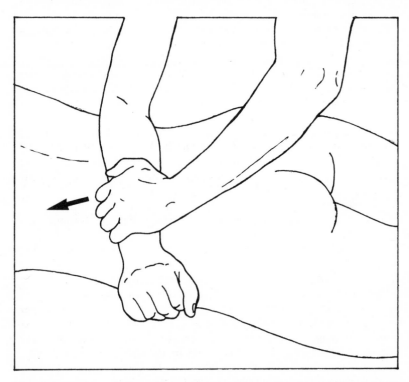

The forearm rub—starting with your arm at the center of your friend's back above the buttocks, move upward and outward (see arrow). Be sure not to put pressure directly on the spine.

Lay the fleshy part of your forearm above your friend's buttocks so that it extends across her entire back at a right angle to her spine. Clench your fist to strengthen your arm muscle and grasp the arm with your other hand so that you can lean into it and increase the pressure. Now, slide the arm upward and outward, toward the far shoulder. Move very slowly. Slide back lightly and repeat, then move to your friend's opposite side and do the step again. (Three repetitions.)

3. *Thumb Friction.* Achy tightness in the latissimus dorsi often occurs in the mid- to lower back where the muscle attaches to connective tissue, called lumbodorsal fascia. This tissue forms a kite shape from the tip of the spine to the midpoint of the back. (The spine, continuing to the skull, looks like the kite's tail.) Prod with your thumbs near the spine on the lower half of the back and you'll find the point where the softer muscle tissue gives way to tougher outward-flaring fascia.

Find the lowest point, just above the ilium, where the muscle and fascia join. Place a thumb at that spot on each side of the back, press firmly, and move your thumbs in circular motions, left thumb clockwise and right counterclockwise. Slide upward along the connecting line and repeat. Continue the motion all the way to the neck. (Two repetitions.) Slide back to the buttocks.

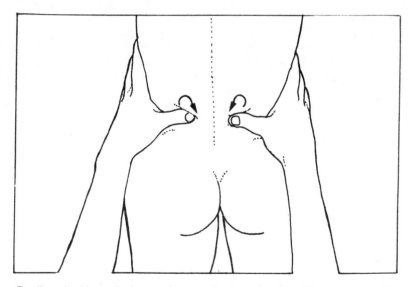

The ilium, that bone that spreads across the lower back and becomes your hip, is where to begin thumb friction. Press firmly and use small, circular motions as illustrated. Slide the thumbs to the next position and repeat to the shoulders.

The Buttocks

Whenever you run or walk or climb steps, one set of muscles repeatedly contracts to bring your legs back under you. In fact, although most people ignore them, they do just about as much work as any other leg muscles when you exercise. They're known as the gluteus maximus (the major buttock muscle), and the gluteus medius (which originates at the ilium, the large hipbone that supports your upper body). Contrary to popular opinion, the primary function of the buttocks muscles is not for sitting.

In modern life, most of us stress the buttocks muscles sporadically. During the week, we're sedentary. We drive to work, sit at a desk or bench or stand at a work table, drive home, and spend the night sitting and sleeping. On the weekend, we might do outdoor things—walk, run, chop wood, play sports. The gluteals are so strong that they can deal with such stresses, but not efficiently. Waste products accumulate between the tissue cells. There are minor tears of muscle tissue. Monday morning, we rarely feel the discomfort in the buttocks. Instead, the pain is *referred*. The symptom you feel might be lower back pain. So it makes sense that an adequate massage of the buttocks frequently eliminates a referred ache in the back.

That's just one of the special benefits of buttock massage. It will also give your friend a beautiful psychological high, which is the purpose of all massage. A thorough buttocks massage is a wonderful conclusion to general massage, and will leave your friend with a warm, peaceful, radiant feeling.

1. *Transition to Buttocks.* Sweep your hands lightly outward across the crest of the ilium until your fingers curve around the hips, then slide down each side until your hands rest on the bottom of the gluteus maximus. Your fingers should be pointing outward and slightly upward. Slide slowly over the buttocks toward the waist with very light pressure, your hands encompassing the buttocks and gently squeezing the muscles inward.

When you reach your friend's waist, slide outward to the sides and downward to the starting position.

Repeat this light stroke twice. Now, do it again, but this time lean into it, increasing the pressure with the heels of your hands. Be sure to keep them far enough apart to avoid putting pressure on the spine, and make sure you press the buttocks together as you proceed. (Two repetitions.)

2. **Heel Rub.** When the buttocks muscles are tightened, hollows —or dimples—appear at each side. As your friend rests on the table, these hollows might not be noticeable, but they are easy enough to feel. Use a sliding stroke to find that area on one side.

Now, place your open hand in the hollow, fingers pointing toward the spine. Rest your other hand on top of the first, press firmly, and move your hand in a circle. This is a compression stroke, not a sliding stroke, so your hand shouldn't move against the skin—the skin should move against the underlying tissue. Do three lingering circles and then move your hand farther up the hollow and repeat. (Repeat this step on the opposite side.)

3. **Heel Vibration.** Standing on one side of your friend, reach across to the opposite side and place the palm of your hand across his thighbone. The heel of your hand should be resting on the gluteus medius, and if you slide your hand toward you, you'll feel the bulge of the gluteus maximus. This is a sensitive area where tension accumulates, and you can do your friend a lot of good by massaging it with two strokes. I suggest you do both on one side, then both on the other.

On the first stroke, apply moderate pressure with the heel of your hand, and rub back and forth rapidly, making the muscle tremble. Continue for at least 30 seconds, moving slowly higher, until your fingers touch the hipbone. (Three repetitions.)

4. **Two-Hand Kneading.** Lay both hands on the gluteus maximus where it dips into the hollow that you've just been vibrating. Your fingers should wrap around the muscle and into the hollow, whereas your thumbs should be extended and pointing toward each other, about an inch apart.

Now squeeze the muscle between your thumb and fingers. When you have a bunch of muscle gathered in both hands, press the hands toward each other to form a bubble of muscle. Slowly relax the squeeze. (Three repetitions for each side.)

5. **Forearm Rub.** This is the same step that you used on the back. It involves the fleshy part of your forearm while your fist is clenched. Begin the stroke just above the knee joint by placing your forearm on the huge hamstring muscle of the thigh. Your hand should be on the outer side of your friend's body, your arm at a 45° angle with the leg, your elbow pointing toward your friend's other knee.

Press hard along the center of the thigh. As you reach the buttocks, keep the pressure over *muscle* rather than *bone*. Move upward and inward. Stop before reaching the spine. (One repetition for each side.)

You've come a long way since first touching your friend's feet. Your friend perhaps has never known such contentment as he or she is feeling right now. You're approaching the final step: ending the massage.

Concluding Strokes

In some respects, a massage is like a novel. When you've read the final word, the lasting impression will be determined neither by the beginning nor the middle, but by how satisfying the ending was. It's the same with massage.

1. *Whole-Body Slide.* End the massage with a gentle whole-body sliding motion. Here's the technique that I often use:

Slide both hands lightly along the spine to the neck, being sure to move very slowly. Massage the neck with your fingertips for a while, then slide along the shoulders and, with open hands, down the sides of the back to the hips. Slide both hands over the buttocks to the thighs—and stop, just resting your hands on the upper thighs. Move very slowly to the inside of the knees—and stop. Move slowly to the ankles, massage the tendons there between thumbs and forefingers. Stop, just holding the tissue there for several seconds. Then slide your hands over the feet. (Three repetitions.)

2. *Wash-down.* If you've used so much lubricant that you must remove some, end with a gentle wash-down. Some people prefer an alcohol rub. I prefer a warm, soapy washcloth. By now your friend's body should be like a musical instrument to you, and you should be the experienced and sensitive musician. If that's the case, you can rely on your own instincts and conclude with the talent in your own hands. It might seem right to linger on the back, on the buttocks, or legs. Perhaps there are still muscles that need special attention—gentle striking with the fingertips, kneading, or just caressing.

You'll become really good at classical massage not merely by learning the techniques discussed in these pages but by something at least equally important—learning to be spontaneous. As I've said earlier, the key to giving your friend all that massage can offer is in listening to your hands as they communicate with his or her body. They'll tell you when to linger, and when to move on. They'll tell you when to knead instead of sliding, when to strike instead of using compression.

Don't be afraid to use your imagination, even inventing your own strokes. When it comes to massaging your friend's body, no one is more expert than you.

CHAPTER SIX

SPECIAL USES FOR CLASSICAL MASSAGE

Beauty

Clothes protect your body from many environmental pollutants, but they don't protect your face. The sulphur, lead, and other chemicals spewed from vehicle exhausts attack it. Dust settles in your pores. You *feel* the dirt. You *see* it accumulate. It's no coincidence that your face shows age faster than the rest of your body. Over time, the skin begins to sag. It grows dry and wrinkled. But classical massage can retard this process, and sometimes even reverse it.

What's more, it can relieve the stress that creates age lines and a haggard appearance. The increased circulation from a good beauty massage will bring added oxygen and nutrients to the skin. And when cleansing is part of a massage for beauty, dry, lifeless skin disappears and only vibrant, healthy skin remains.

CLEANSING

Massage for beauty should begin with cleansing, starting with a deep-down, pore-opening, circulation-stimulating facial.

The most enduring method of softening dry skin and opening the pores is to apply hot towels. Select small ones. When folded in half, they should fit neatly from your friend's hairline to her neck.

If the water is so hot that you can't wring out the towel without burning your hand, it's certainly too hot for your friend's face. Abbott and Costello entertained us with barber shop scenes in which the customer became the victim of hot towel tortures, but your friend won't laugh at being burned. The towel should be comfortably warm when applied, and because it will cool in two or three minutes, a second towel should be warming at arm's length for immediate replacement.

The warming device I prefer is an electric slow-cooking pot. I've also used a portable electric plate to heat water in a cooking pot. Unless you've set up a massage table in your kitchen, the ordinary stove is no good—you'll spend all your time running back and forth instead of concentrating on your friend's face.

Here's a good system for changing towels without exposing the face to the cool air:

Lay the warm towel, folded in half, on your friend's neck. With your left thumb and forefinger, grasp the lower left corner of the cool towel (the one to be removed) and the upper left corner of the warm one. Grasp the corresponding corners with your right thumb and forefinger. Pull both towels taut, lift the towels and slide them upward, gathering the cool towel with your remaining fingers as you proceed. When the warm towel is in place, remove the cool one entirely.

You can make the hot towel even more effective—and stimulating—by adding a heat-producing oil to the water. Pure oil of wintergreen does nicely if your friend finds the aroma pleasant. Wintergreen is the heat-producing ingredient in many rubbing compounds. You can buy the pure oil in any well-stocked pharmacy.

Add about half a teaspoon to 4 cups of water. Much more than that can cause sensitive facial skin to burn. The oil will float on the surface of the water until the water begins to simmer. Then, by stirring, you can break up the globules.

Allow the water to cool until you can soak the towel and wring it out without burning yourself. Wring the towel thoroughly, and tell your friend to keep her eyes closed—even extremely diluted concentrations of wintergreen in the eyes can be painful, if not dangerous.

If wintergreen isn't for you or your friend, perhaps eucalyptus oil is. That, too, gives a warm, tingling feeling—and also must be kept out of the eyes.

An alternative to oils and the heat they produce is herbs. Just about every herb has probably been used in facials, and although they have limited physical benefits, they add a pleasant fragrance.

Or add half a teaspoon of any spice you enjoy smelling. My own favorite is cloves. (Use whole cloves rather than powdered, about six of them to 4 cups of water.) If you *do* use a powdered herb or spice, be sure to end the facial with a thorough washing with warm water and a gentle soap before moving on to the facial massage.

The pores of your friend's face are now open. Dust and bacteria are now exposed. Dead skin cells have been loosened. It's time to cleanse the face, either with soap and warm water or a warm, damp towel. Make sure that your own hands, the towel, and the water you're using are clean—don't use the water containing oils or herbs.

Begin at the hairline and, with a very light stroke, as though powdering the face, cleanse the forehead from the center outward on each side. You need to use only the index and second finger of one hand, the towel wrapped around the fingers. Rinse the towel frequently—at least twice while cleansing the forehead.

Continue cleansing the entire face. Pay special attention to the outside corners of the eyes, the fleshy parts of the nostrils, the cleft of the chin, and the ears—any crevices where dirt or dead skin cells are likely to accumulate.

When you're finished, your friend's face should feel tingling and warm, those facial muscles as ready as they can be for your massage.

THE BRUSH TECHNIQUE

Another effective way to remove dead skin cells, cleanse the pores, and stimulate circulation—all while giving your friend a very special experience—is to use a brush. The trick is to get the right brush—a toothbrush will feel like sandpaper, as will most alternatives. The ideal is the old barber's shaving lather brush. The bristles form a soft, round puff. You can still buy these brushes in stores that specialize in shaving accessories.

You can also use a small paintbrush—the 1-inch size—from your local hardware store. Make sure the bristles are natural (not nylon) and very soft.

Follow the same pattern that you used for cleansing, beginning at the forehead and working to the chin. Use a light, circular stroke at least three times in each area, overlapping so that the entire face is brushed.

Avoid causing irritation. Also, it isn't necessary to brush near the eyes and risk poking beneath the eyelid. Conclude by cleansing with a damp, warm towel.

I don't recommend a powder or lotion when using a brush. The lotion obviously gets to be a gooey mess in the bristles and accomplishes nothing. Although talcum powder is pleasant and lets the bristles slide easily, it counteracts the purpose of the brush massage in the first place: to help remove impurities from the pores and scrape off dead skin cells. If you want to use a brush simply for the pleasure it gives (and it does), apply an astringent first to close the pores.

ASTRINGENTS

After you've cleaned the skin and pores, it's time to close them up again. You can do that in several ways.

One is water. Ice water will promptly tighten the skin—but it might also give your friend an unpleasant surprise.

Alcohol is the most popular astringent. It also makes the skin feel cool (although very briefly), unless the brush massage caused tiny nicks, in which case alcohol can cause painful stings.

The tannic acid in tea makes an excellent astringent. I use instant tea, four spoons to a cup of tepid water together with a teaspoon of lemon juice. Tell your friend to keep her eyes closed —the lemon juice is an irritant—and apply the solution lavishly. Allow your friends face to dry in the air awhile before dabbing it with a soft cloth.

The Facial Massage

1. *Forehead Slide.* If you've ever watched an athlete under enormous stress, you might have noticed the blood vessels bulging on his forehead. These vessels are large and dramatic, and they play a major role in facial circulation. Because the upper forehead in particular gets so little exercise, this area can benefit greatly from the "passive exercise" of massage.

Standing beside your friend, rest the palms of your hands over her eyes, thumbs together on her forehead, thumb tips pressing the hairline. Keep your fingers closed, turned outward and resting on the temples.

Using firm pressure, slide the thumbs out toward the sides of the forehead. Simultaneously, let your palms glide gently over the eyelids. (Five repetitions.)

2. *Face Mash.* You really won't be mashing anybody's face with this stroke, but it's a memorable title, and it does describe a technique that exercises the largest muscles of the face.

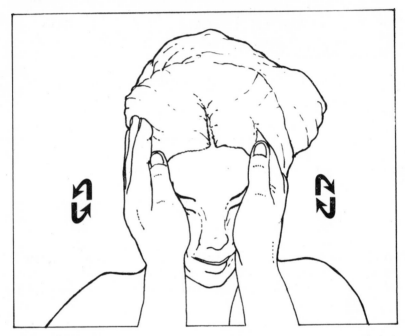

The face mash is a friction stroke—your hands don't move across the skin but cause the skin to move against underlying tissue. Move your entire hand, including fingers, so that all of the face is passively exercised.

Cup your hands over your friend's cheekbones, your fingers together and extending to the sides of your friend's forehead. Move both hands in a circular compression motion, the left hand clockwise, the right counterclockwise.

As the hands move toward each other, the fingers will press forehead tissue together and the palms will do the same to the lips and cheeks. As the hands move down and outward, facial tissue will be stretched. If your friend's face shows any sign of tension, you'll see the stress vanish before your eyes as you apply this stroke. (Three repetitions.)

3. *Crow's-Feet Rub.* Crow's-feet—the lines at the outer corners of your eyes that children never have and older people almost always do—bother a great many people. That's unfortunate because these

lines usually attest to character. They come from frequent squinting of the eyes in laughter or weeping, and sometimes just from tension. Eventually, the creasing usually becomes permanent.

I say *usually* because these lines can actually be massaged away. Place your thumbs over them and move them in a semicircular pattern, using enough pressure to flatten the lines out. (Continue until they disappear.)

Done regularly, the creases will become significantly less obvious.

If getting rid of these crow's-feet is the main purpose of the massage, apply a skin moisturizer to the creases, and rub gently. Most moisturizers will permeate the skin, sort of like tucking a tiny pillow beneath this loose area. Once the moisturizer is absorbed, dab the area with an astringent to tighten the skin. Obviously, keep the astringent out of your friend's eyes.

The combined effect of the whole procedure is this. You've ironed the wrinkles out of the skin with your thumbs, supported the skin with an underlying cushion of moisturizer, and then tightened the skin with alcohol. These effects will last only a short time, but during that period, those permanent press creases will lose their permanence. Now, if your friend makes a habit of totally relaxing her face for several minutes twice a day, and/or rubs away the crow's-feet daily, they'll be far less of a problem.

RELAXATION STROKES

Stress lines almost always occur because we carry our daily tensions in those overworked muscles of our face. You can see it for yourself during a bus or subway ride by studying the faces of those sitting across the aisle from you. You can tell by the muscle tension who has serious problems, and by the completely flaccid facial muscles who has given up.

Unrelieved facial tension is the enemy of youthful looks. The following strokes are designed specifically to help facial muscles to relax.

4. *Ear Caress.* Place the palms of your hands over your friend's ears and stroke in a circular movement, moving your fingers over the scalp above the ears. (Continue for about a minute or until your friend seems noticeably more relaxed than when you started the stroke.)

5. *The Puppy Pet.* Dogs can be virtually hypnotized with this stroke, and it's a wonderful relaxer for humans, too. Standing behind your friend's head, bring one hand to rest across her fore-

head low enough so the side of your little finger rests at the bridge of her nose. Stroke slowly and lightly upward, and as the first hand moves across the hairline and onto the scalp, begin the same stroke with your other hand. (Continue for at least 1 minute.)

6. *Jowl Knead.* The cheekbone, base of the ear, and tip of the chin form a triangle of cheek flesh that responds well to gentle kneading between the thumbs and first fingers. Start at the lips and work upward along the cheekbone to the ears. Tug the ear-lobes and knead around them, then move down along the jawbone to the chin. Don't knead over the chin itself—it's too bony.

As you knead, squeeze the tissue into hills of flesh that run parallel to the nose—top to bottom of the face rather than left to right. That produces a much more pleasant feeling. (Three repetitions.)

The Scalp Massage

First, you should know the truth. There's no evidence that scalp massage will help hair to grow on a bald spot; it won't combat grayness.

Scalp massage *will* stimulate circulation, prompt the oil-secreting glands to become more active, and remove dry, scaly skin—dandruff. Dry and damaged hair can be remarkably transformed by regular scalp massage.

Begin with the strokes for the scalp described on pages 45–46. Thereafter, follow up with any—or all—of the following strokes. The goal of these techniques is simply to make sure that every centimeter of the scalp is massaged vigorously enough to stimulate the capillary circulation, invigorate oil glands, and remove dry skin. It doesn't matter whether you use the index and second finger (as one expert instructs), your thumbs (as another advocates), or all your fingers and the palm of your hand in the bargain. And it doesn't matter if you go left to right, right to left, front to back, or back to front, as long as you vigorously massage the entire scalp.

My own preference is to use the heels of my hands because it's easier to sustain pressure with them than with my fingers. I begin a circular compression motion at the hairline—compression because it eliminates the possibility of pulling the hair away from the skin; with·compression, hair and skin move together against underlying tissue.

I start in the center of the forehead. Following a series of circular motions I slide an inch or so farther up the scalp and repeat. The direction is along the center of the scalp to the back of the neck, along the underside of the scalp over the ears to the temples, and to the forehead. Then, once again I start back across the scalp, this time with my hands farther apart.

Following this pattern, I eliminate the possibility of pushing the hair against its natural grain, which is about as painful as tearing it out by the roots. When the massage is finished, a nice thing to do is to place the fingers of both hands on your friend's scalp as though they were spider legs and your hands the spider's body. Now, simply scratch the head rapidly and all over.

End the scalp massage by rinsing the hair in tepid water. It isn't necessary to use a shampoo, but if you feel you must, make sure it's mild.

There are no special massage techniques for beautifying the body. You *can* increase blood circulation and nutrition to specific areas of the body and reduce accumulation of waste products there through massage. The techniques are exactly the same as those you learned in Chapter Five.

Keep in mind that many of us appear to have less beautiful bodies than we do because we don't *feel* beautiful. As a result, we don't carry ourselves proudly. We allow our postures to sag. Many times I've massaged friends' bodies "for beauty," and later they have appeared truly more beautiful because the massage has made them feel that way. That's because beauty often is limited not by nature but by self-image. We all know of women who are stoop-shouldered because they still harbor the adolescent embarrassment of ample breasts, adult men who still behave as though they are awkward and gangly. Others feel too fat or too skinny or mis-shapen.

I know a 40-year-old woman who for the first 35 years of her life could not conquer the shame of being fat. In fact, although she had been overweight as a teenager, she had developed a full but beautiful figure by her mid-twenties. Yet, she would never date, because "it might lead to undressing, and I just couldn't let any-one see me like this."

Six months with a psychiatrist didn't help. Then, her best friend persuaded her to accept a massage. After three weeks of whole-body massage, the woman developed a much more positive self-image. When she looked in the mirror, it was as though she were seeing herself for the first time. She thought she was as beautiful as the massages made her feel.

Good hands tell the truth about our bodies, stressing the natural grace and beauty that exists in all of us.

Sports

For the athlete, massage contributes significantly to conditioning and performance. It's more than a matter of winning and losing—it can make the difference between staying in the game and being sidelined with injuries.

The same is true for anyone who is physically active, whether he jogs, swims, or cycles daily or, as is frequently the case, is sedentary six days a week, then plays racquetball or some other strenuous game on the seventh. In fact, physically active people will find the healing effects of sports massage particularly welcome.

There are four basic categories of sports massage, and each is important in helping to achieve his or her maximum capability:

- The conditioning massage
- The warm-up massage
- The post-activity massage
- The therapeutic massage

The Conditioning Massage

Conditioning massage, should be given 24 hours before the athlete is to perform in competition. The goal is *total relaxation.*

First the athlete should take a brisk needle shower, starting with warm water, then switching to cool—about 80°F.

The athlete should lie on his stomach, and you should concentrate on the massive back muscles. Once these are relaxed, the rest of the body tends to relax as well. Begin with sweeping but superficial slide strokes over the entire back, then add moderate and finally firm pressure.

Kneading with both hands, as described on page 54 will also be effective, but avoid striking and pinching strokes, cold hands, or anything else that will stimulate the muscles to tighten in the slightest.

You can't give a conditioning massage by the clock. The massage is complete not when a clock says so but when the athlete is totally relaxed.

You may go a step further when the athlete is completely relaxed, and it will pay dividends the next day: Devote your attention to the muscles he or she will use in the competition itself. Most sports put the greatest demand on the legs, so, usually, after sliding down to the feet, you can massage both front and back of each leg separately, using the strokes described on pages 28–34.

Keep in mind that the gluteal muscles, or buttocks, function as leg muscles in running and jumping sports and should be given as much attention as the other leg muscles.

The conditioning massage is definitely not whole-body. It's specific to the back and the muscles most involved in athletic performance, and its goal is to relax and refresh those muscles.

Studies have shown that massage can lift conditioned muscles to an even higher level of excellence, significantly increasing the amount of work they can do while decreasing recovery time. That's especially important in sports such as football, where effort is intense but sporadic.

An additional benefit: Well-massaged muscles are less likely to spasm, cramp, or tear.

Following the conditioning massage, the athlete should rest on the massage table for at least 20 minutes, then take a warm shower before dressing or sleeping.

The Warm-Up Massage

This is given shortly before competition and is immediately followed by the athlete's routine warm-up exercises. It benefits the athlete in many ways—and sometimes the effects can be dramatic.

PRE-GAME JITTERS

Many athletes, like thoroughbred race horses, are so highstrung that much of the energy that should be going into competition is wasted in nervousness. Heart rate, blood pressure, and basal metabolism all increase, using up the most readily available energy sources—just the ones the athlete will need during hard competition.

What's more, when the body grows tense from nervousness, most major muscle groups tighten. Those muscles are doing work —although they aren't accomplishing anything. Simply by being tense, or contracting, even if only subtly, the muscles are using more oxygen and giving off more lactic acid as waste than they would if they were completely relaxed. The result is that the athlete enters competition with muscles already on the road to exhaustion and his or her instant energy supply dwindling.

MUSCLE STRETCHING

Like the stretch exercises in every good warm-up routine, massage coaxes the muscles into greater flexibility—but it does it in a more subtle way.

Most of us have known the occasional morning when even climbing out of bed seems to require too much effort. Our bodies don't actually ache, and it's nothing we can pinpoint precisely, but each move seems to require so much *effort*. We say our muscles are *stiff*.

Athletes face the same problem, usually the result of shortened muscles in constant combat with each other. Here's what I mean:

As you know, our muscles do their work by contracting, or shortening. For each muscle, there's an opposing one to produce an opposite movement. To lift your leg straight out in front of you, for example, you'd use the rectus and quadriceps of the front of the upper thigh. But to extend your leg outward behind you like a ballerina, these muscles would have to *relax* while the hamstring muscles *contract*.

When muscles shorten, they will *not* relax as much as they should. To do its job, the opposing muscle must not only fight the ordinary forces of gravity and body weight, but now it must also combat the resistance of the shortened opposing muscle. The result is that all the muscles involved quickly grow weary. It's that sense of our bodies fighting within themselves that makes the effort to get up in the morning so disagreeable for some of us. Only after we've moved around for a while and loosened up these muscles do we feel comfortable.

Some athletes can move quickly into a warm-up routine that includes muscle stretching, but others—especially in cold weather —run the risk of tearing muscles or suffering cramps by hasty warm-up exercises. Massage can stretch these stiff muscles, increase their temperature and circulation, and prepare the athlete safely for his warm-up routine.

THE STROKES

For the warm-up massage, use the same relaxation strokes as described for the conditioning massage above. Generally, the warm-up massage is intended to do just that—to warm up the body. Warm muscles tend to relax, and relaxed muscles are more efficient processors of nutrients and oxygen. (The idea that a hot sauna is a great way to relax is no myth.)

Whole-body sliding strokes are great for stimulating heat and blood flow. These should start superficially but quickly build to deep strokes. Use a lubricant for deep stroking so that you don't pull the hair out of the athlete's body as a result of excessive rubbing against the skin. I prefer not to use a lotion with a heat-producing ingredient in either the conditioning or warm-up massage, for I suspect that this artificial sedative .to the muscles can be excessive; when the muscles are called on to work, they might respond just a slight bit sluggishly—and that can make the difference between victory and defeat.

The Post-Activity Massage

The time for including wintergreen or eucalyptus or rubbing lotion is *after* competition, when it's important that the extremely worked muscles don't tighten. The first order of business is to make sure that those muscles don't chill and contract in a protective spasm. This should be a matter of priority, particularly in cold weather.

If a shower is really necessary before post-activity massage— and it usually isn't (perspiration is a rather good, although socially frowned-upon lubricant)—the water should be warm or tepid, but not cold. And the massage room should be 72°F or warmer.

Apart from keeping the muscles warm, don't worry about tightened muscles. Ordinarily, these muscles are going to relax now that they've worked themselves to exhaustion. Instead, the techniques you use should help to move waste products that accumulate between the cells of hard-working muscles out of those spaces and toward the bloodstream. Studies have shown that the proper massage after exercise can dramatically reduce the time it takes muscles to recuperate.

That means that your strokes should always be *from* the extremities toward the heart. An entire arm or leg might be "milked" by using both hands to squeeze a large muscle, one hand for a smaller one. Keep thinking in terms of emptying a tube of toothpaste— envision the muscle being wrung out.

For example, let's assume we're massaging the upper thigh. Standing next to your friend, lay both hands flat and side by side on the thigh. Begin by squeezing the lowest fingers of your lower hand—the one closest to the knee—pressing the leg muscle into the palm of your hand. Continue to squeeze with the middle fingers and thumb while sliding the hand upward until both your hands touch.

Resume the squeezing with your upper hand—thumb and first few fingers—while the lower hand relaxes. Finally, contract the last fingers of the upper hand, then slide this hand upward to the groin. (Three repetitions, followed by a deep slide from the knee to hip.)

The Therapeutic Massage

A day or two after strenuous physical activity most athletes, no matter how well conditioned, will feel sore and stiff. Sometimes it lasts for only a couple of days, but a week of aches and pains isn't that unusual.

There are two theories to explain this condition. One is that lactic acid, the waste product that results from the burning of great amounts of oxygen during exercise, accumulates between the muscle cells and, like grains of sand, causes irritation and pain when the muscle fibers move. The second theory is that during exercise tiny muscle fibers tear, and until they heal they cause minor pain.

In either case, the strokes described for post-activity massage should be adapted for the specific muscle groups that are painful. The strokes should be done *very* slowly—20 seconds or more for an entire arm, 30 seconds or more for a leg.

MUSCLE CRAMPS

Physicians don't know for sure what causes muscle cramps, but they definitely know what a muscle cramp is (and so do you, if you've ever had one). Either because of a deficiency in the enzyme cholinesterase, which "tells" the muscle to relax when the brain so orders, or a blood deficiency to the muscle, or excess nervous stimulation, or some other reason, the cramped muscle simply contracts with the tenacity of a bullterrier who has sunk his teeth into a trespasser's leg. The contraction is so violent that it causes significant pain, and the irony is that what seems like the natural thing—favoring the cramped limb by protecting it from motion—is exactly the wrong approach.

The first thing to do when a cramp seems to be coming on is to flex or stretch the tightening muscle. If it is caught soon enough, the cramp will disappear before it ever becomes painful.

If the muscle is already severely cramped, the victim probably won't be able to stretch it by himself. That's when massage comes in. First, you should gently but firmly stretch the cramped limb. If the cramp is in the foot, the toes will curve downward, toward the sole. Grasp them firmly and bend them back with one hand while holding the heel in the other. When the pain eases, use your thumb to gently massage the irritated muscle. A heat-generating ointment such as Ben-Gay will help the muscle to relax.

A pain in the calf can be eased by tilting the entire foot so that the toes are pointing up toward the knee and the heel down and away from the body.

Hamstring cramps can be relieved by having the victim lie on his back while you lift the affected leg upward with the knee straight, the toes of that foot bent toward the shinbone. Press the leg back as far as necessary while the victim keeps his knee straight.

SPRAINS

First, be sure the injury is a sprain and not a fracture which needs medical attention.

Cold compresses will ease the pain and reduce the amount of fluid that would otherwise accumulate at the injury site. The goal of massage is to disperse these excess fluids by gently stroking them from the sprain location toward the heart. Alternate with strokes from the heart toward the injury to ensure good circulation and nutrition. Be exceedingly gentle, and if you notice any redness developing—a sign of infection—stop immediately.

Muscle and ligament tears respond very well to massage, apparently because circulation is improved. The added nutrients thus obtained speed the healing process.

Finally, localized muscle injuries can often be dramatically relieved through a technique known as *deep friction massage*. If you massage an athlete regularly, you'll do him or her a great favor by studying the section on deep friction massage—carefully.

Sensual Pleasure

In this section, you'll learn some special techniques that will enhance and intensify the sexual bond between two people. Massage, you see, not only feels wonderful, but is a way of focusing on instincts and desires, and creating an environment of intimacy and pleasure-giving. It's also a way of learning, or relearning, how to touch each other.

THE ATMOSPHERE

It's difficult to give or receive sensual massage if somewhere in the back of your mind you know a telephone may ring, the kids may burst into the room, or company may knock on the door. Most people relax best in familiar surroundings. So, take the phone off the hook, send the kids to an understanding relative or friend, and select a day and time when visits aren't likely. It might be worthwhile to take a vacation day from work while the children are in school and spend the whole time with your husband or wife. On the other hand, if you prefer spontaneity, it might be best to just let things happen and risk the interruptions.

Choose a room that's warm and has a cozy atmosphere. Eliminate glaring lights.

Soft music enhances relaxation for some people, but for others it's a distraction. You might begin with appropriate music and turn it off as the massage progresses.

Showering together is a pleasant prelude to sensual massage, particularly because our society seems bent on eliminating all traces of natural body fragrance in favor of synthetic odors (although body odors are primary sex attractants among animals and insects). For many people, nonetheless, cleanliness is essential to intimacy, and the surest way to know that your partner's body is clean is to wash it yourself while he or she washes you.

A warm shower also fosters relaxation. For those who might find the intimacy of massage embarrassing and tension-producing, a shared shower breaks the ice.

Although you and your lover should feel free to wash all parts of each other's bodies, if appropriate, the shower should *not* be genitally centered; otherwise it will decrease the effect of the sensual massage.

Finally, there's the question of whether or not to use a massage table for sensual massage. Although there's no doubt that you can give a much more thorough massage with a table, thoroughness is not the objective here—intimacy is. I prefer a firm bed. If your bed sags, put a board under the mattress, and protect the mattress with a rubber or plastic waterproof sheet. Above that, use a covering of your choice—linen, leather—or satin, if the room is really warm.

STROKES

The purpose of a sensual massage is, obviously, not the same as other general massage. Usually, one of the highest compliments your friend can pay you is to fall asleep when you are massaging him, but that's not the response you want in sensual massage. A general massage should produce total relaxation, but sensual massage seeks *limited* relaxation: The cares of the outside world slip away as you focus your partner's attention on his or her own body. To concentrate that attention you must use strokes we've not discussed before, strokes that say, in effect, "Notice this part of your body, how it feels when it's touched like this; doesn't it feel good?"

Think of the strokes in sensual massage as caresses. You're petting your partner, not achieving physiological benefits as in other forms of massage—although, hopefully, there'll be a significant increase in his or her heart rate and oxygen consumption.

Your Fingers. You can do most of the strokes using just the balls of your fingers in a light, teasing stroke. Slide the fingers toward you only—if you also use your fingertips in an away stroke, there will be greater pressure, and friction, and the difference can distract your friend.

The backs of your fingers can be used for a pleasant away stroke, however. Lay the entire backs of your fingers against the large muscles of your friend's body—legs, buttocks, back, chest, and abdomen—and use a flicking movement, as though brushing crumbs from your lap.

You can also bend your fingers at the joints closest to the tips and do an away stroke with the backs of your fingernails.

Fingernails. The classic *Kama Sutra,* the ancient Hindu love manual by Vatsyayana, elevates the fingernail to the status of a virtual sex organ, actually distinguishing lovers by the quality of their fingernails. Vatsyayana describes eight techniques for using the nails, and writes, "The parts of the body on which these caresses should be perpetrated are: the armpit, the throat, the breast, the lips, the jaghana (abdomen), and the thighs."

The technique we're interested in is the *churit-nakhadana,* which causes the partner to shiver "till the woman's body-hair bristles up, and a shudder passes all over the limbs."

Use the fingernails in all the places Vatsyayana described (the armpits can be a particular delight if you are not so gentle as to tickle your partner)—and anywhere else the stroke seems appropriate. Your nails should not be sharp, ragged, or pointed. As to how much pressure you should use, your own common sense will dictate that. Many people are sexually stimulated by a degree of roughness, and no harm's done by leaving red lines in the wake of your fingernails if it delights your friend. Others find that kind of treatment painful rather than erotic, though, so it's up to you to find out what your friend enjoys.

Hands. Some strokes can be done best with the whole hand. In sensual massage, the touch should always be very light. For something different and special, try wearing soft leather or velvet gloves. Some people are not affected by these items and would prefer to feel flesh on flesh, but for those who enjoy them, leather or velvet gloves are ecstasy.

Lips, Tongue, and Teeth. Shaykh Nafzawi advises in *The Perfumed Garden:* "You will excite her by kissing her cheeks, sucking her lips and nibbling at her breasts. You will lavish kisses on her navel and titillate the lower parts. Bite at her arms and neglect no part of her body . . ."

Although the techniques I'll describe are usually performed with hands or fingers, many can be adapted. For example, few experiences are so erotic as having your neck and ears caressed by another's tongue. It's probably instinctive to caress the breasts with the lips. And it's a beautiful experience to nibble gently the inner arms and thighs.

Hair. Unless your hair is very short, you can give your partner a wonderful feeling by caressing his or her entire body by whisking your hair over it. Move slowly, as though your hair were fingers, and follow the same directions you would for hand or finger strokes. Keep the weight of your head off your friend—let the hair do the caressing—and avoid your friend's face; the irritation of having hair in eyes, nose, and mouth distracts from any sensual delights.

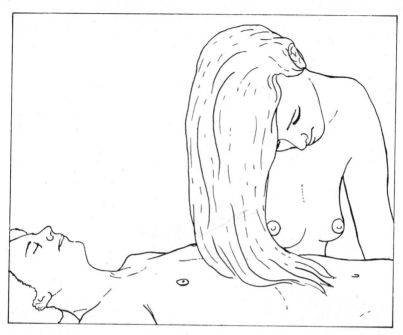

Long hair slowly caressing one's body can be uniquely stimulating—like the touch of a feather but more satisfying because it can tingle the entire abdomen in a single stroke. There is also something sensual about the fragrance of human hair for most men and women. The only caution: keep your hair out of your friend's face.

The Sensual Massage

The following should serve as a guide, not a bible. Adapt it to your circumstances, and always trust your natural inclination. We'll assume that your friend is lying on his or her abdomen to begin.

1. *Calf Slide.* Begin at the Achilles tendon above the heel and slide up along the inside of the calf to your partner's knee joint. Linger with soft, circular strokes in this area behind the knee— it's highly sensitive. Slide down along the center and outer part of

the calf to the ankle. (As in all strokes to follow, let your instincts dictate the number of repetitions.)

2. *Thigh/Buttocks Slide.* Begin by straddling your friend's legs. Trace a line from the knee joint along the inner thighs. If you're using your entire hands for the stroke, lay them fully on the hamstring, and allow your thumbs to trace the inner thighs. At the buttocks, apply firm but gentle pressure upward toward the spine, the thumbs still tracing the inner extremes of the gluteal muscles.

Ease back to very light pressure as you reach the hipbones, slide outward to the sides and along the sides to the knee joints.

Although the thumbs might brush the genitals during this stroke, it's important at this point not to linger there. Heightened desire arises from anticipation, and the sexually wise lover knows that teasing, flirting, and the uncertainty of fulfillment all play a major part in heightening our sexual interest. In sensual massage per se, genital contact should be avoided, or at most, fleeting.

3. *The Back Scratch.* The easiest way to get most people to purr like kittens is to gently scratch their backs. Long strokes, beginning at the base of the neck near the spine and extending to the ilium, or hipbone, are usually the most satisfying, but use any stroke pattern you like—circular, shingling, from the spine outward, or whatever. Just be consistent. The human mind being what it is, your friend will unconsciously want to recognize a pattern in your stroke and relax in it. Variation will be distracting.

The only potential problem with back scratching is that it can be *too* relaxing. You don't want your partner to fall asleep. If you see your friend becoming more relaxed than stimulated, you might want to vary your method for applying the stroke, zigzagging the lines, using open hands with your fingers tracing the sides of the breasts and such.

Some practitioners put great emphasis on massaging the area surrounding the sacrum, the large bone at the base of the spine. They point out—correctly—that a number of nerves leading to the reproductive organs are concentrated in this area, and they claim that these nerves can be stimulated through massage.

I mention this because it can do no harm to massage the sacral area with light to medium pressure, and it might be a pleasant experience for your friend. But the fact is, these nerves are so completely protected by the skeleton that you're unlikely to stimulate them manually.

4. *Hair Stroking.* "One of the best ways of kindling hot desire in a woman is, at the time of rising, softly to hold and handle the

hair . . ." such is the advice offered in *The Hindu Art of Love*. Hair stroking is not scalp massage. It more closely resembles a gentle shampoo without the shampoo.

When your partner has rolled onto his back, kneel at his head. Use the fingers of both hands to comb the hair gently upward toward the top of your friend's head and away from the ears. If the hair is long enough, it can be tugged gently, especially if it can be gathered in a single clump. When this is done properly, it is like a thousand little fingers massaging every part of the scalp.

With your hands cupped, place your fingers on your friend's head and massage with very rapid, tingling movements. Concentrate on the base of the skull and the area around the ears.

Gather the hair and tumble it between your hands.

5. *The Neck Caress.* With one hand at the base of your friend's skull, lift your friend's head. With the other, caress the back of the neck along its entire length on each side of the spine.

Allow your friend's head to rest on the bed again. Using thumbnails only, trace the throat *from* the chest *to* the head on each side of the esophagus. After several repetitions, use your fingers along the sides of the neck in the same stroke.

6. *Ear Stimulation.* There might actually be a physiological reason for the popular maximum, "Blow in his ear and he'll follow you anywhere." The vagus nerve, which extends from the base of the brain to all of the body's extremities, influences the autonomic nervous system—which in turn helps to regulate sexual response. Acupuncturists sometimes insert gold darts or earrings into the ears, to be worn for several weeks or months, on the theory that continuous stimulation of the vagus nerve will restore sexual potency.

If I'm fortunate enough to have my ears stimulated, I prefer not a gold dart but the lips or tongue of a loving friend. If you're the giver of such a treat, try to relax and do what's spontaneous. Feel your friend's delight as though it were happening to you and do what you would like done. Nibble the earlobe with lips and teeth. Trace the ear crevices with your tongue.

Here's a really special modification of the traditional blowing in the ear: Rather than merely blowing, make a "brrrr" sound—as children, we called it giving the raspberries. Allow your lips to vibrate so that the air is expelled in pulsations.

Spend as much time as you can on the ears. Trace them with your fingers, cup them with the palms of your hands, caress them as part of a neck massage. For many people, the ears are the key to wide-open sensual experience.

7. *Abdominal Slide.* From the ears, slide along the throat and across the center of the chest, your fingers pointing toward the pubic bone. As your hands slip beyond the ribs and continue toward the lower abdomen, turn your fingers outward while the heels of your hands remain together. The pressure for the entire stroke should be light, but it should increase slightly as your hands pass over the navel. That helps to increase the amount of blood accumulating in the pubic region.

When you reach the pubic bone, slide your hands outward to the sides and return to the armpits in a slow, feathery stroke. Bring your hands across the top of the chest until they meet beneath the throat, fingers turning toward the pubic bone again. Repeat the entire series.

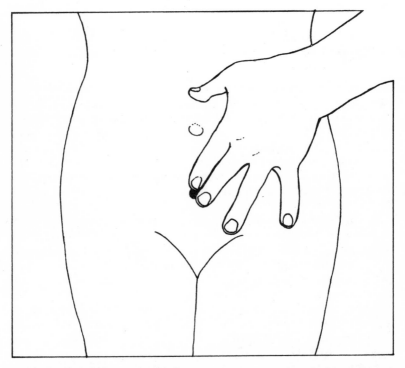

You may not give much credence to the Oriental meridians, but some experimenting will at least make you believe in the "Gate of Origin." Gentle, continuing pressure focusing on upward sliding strokes in this area can actually bring some women to orgasm.

8. *The Lower Abdomen Press*. For thousands of years, Orientals have recognized the significance of the lower abdomen in sexuality. The "gate of origin" as it's called, is located 3 inches below the navel, and stimulating it is believed to help overcome frigidity and impotence. Pressure here directly affects genital circulation.

Begin with any light strokes using your hands, fingers, lips or tongue. The purpose is to focus your friend's attention on this part of his or her body.

Place the palm of your hand just above the pubic bone and increase pressure gradually. Maintain moderate pressure for 10 to 15 seconds, then slowly relax. This stroke should be done only once.

You're still kneeling at your friend's head. With the heel of each hand resting on either side of the navel, your fingers extending to the pubic bone, slide your hands downward (toward your friend's thighs) and inward. Start the stroke with very light pressure and increase to moderate as the heels of your hands reach the pubic bone. Return with the feathery stroke and repeat.

For Men

Regardless of the current popularity of androgyny, many scientific studies show that men and women do not respond in the same way to sexual stimuli—studies show that women prefer subtle love stories, men "hard action." That's as true of sensual massage as it is of pornography. When it comes to massage, women are *generally* more responsive to lingering, gentle stimulation, whereas men prefer a firmer, action-oriented approach.

If your partner is a man, you might find him responding with great pleasure when you use your fingernails for virtually all the massage techniques. If you notice that he reacts positively, continue to use your nails on his abdomen, the insides of his thighs, his sides. How hard should you scratch? If you break the skin, obviously you're scratching too hard. Beyond that, you must read your friend's face and the sounds he makes. Some men will find erotic what others find painful.

If you have long hair, you can give your friend a very special treat by simply brushing it like a handful of feathers over his entire body, head to toe, back and front. Although this is a very gentle sensation, it's loaded with erotic implications and most men delight in it.

Gently pinching the inner thighs, lower abdomen, and buttocks stimulates many men, as does moderate slapping of the buttocks.

For Women

So thoroughly did the Hindus develop the art of sensual massage for women that *The Hindu Art of Love* contains instructions detailing how virtually every part of the body is to be treated—including the right eye, lower lip, left cheek, and big toe. Times and tastes change, of course, and some of these techniques are not likely to be successful today. For example: throat—hug with force. Arm—jerk suddenly and twitch. Breast—rub, twist, and make it very small. Armpit—scratch and tickle.

The Hindus also practiced gentler strokes, however, and some of them remain the epitome of sensual massage even today.

THROAT, FACE, AND EARS

Many men shy away from having their face and throat doted upon at length. It's very likely a cultural reaction—animals show surrender in a fight by exposing their throats to the victors. And men are perhaps culturally conditioned not to surrender, even symbolically and even when the surrender is to love. Regardless of the reason, the fact stands, and most men will enjoy facial play for only a moment, and will tolerate it only a little longer.

Women, on the other hand, have no such inhibitions. Many enjoy having their throats caressed for extended periods with fingers, lips, and tongue. Begin facial strokes with a single finger at the center of the forehead sliding to the temple, tracing the ear, moving along the chin line, to the other ear, temple, and back to the center of the forehead. You can repeat the stroke many times, creating an almost hypnotic effect.

Follow it with a light, circular cheek stroke, using the backs of your fingers. Then, slide to the throat.

THE BREASTS

The male has so thoroughly capsulized the sexuality of females in their breasts that a curious thing has happened to the female psyche as a result. Early in adolescence, girls recognize their breasts as the first public declaration of their womanhood. They're also the first part of the anatomy on which most boys focus their sexual attention. Having the breasts caressed is highly stimulating for most girls at first, but as the years pass, some women find it so commonplace as to be void of excitement. The goal in sensual breast massage is to restore the original ardor that the caress first produced. To do that, you must focus complete attention on the breasts.

Begin by placing a pillow under your partner's back, lifting the breasts high. Straddle her hips. Begin stroking with one or two fingers at the armpits, moving down and inward, just grazing the sides of the breasts and continuing beneath them to the sternum. Return to the armpits, using the backs of your fingers.

On the next stroke, move higher on the breasts, to the sternum, then back to the armpits. Only when your fingers reach the areola (the puckered dark skin surrounding the nipples) should you change your strokes.

Now, circle the areola twice. Open your hand and stroke the outer half of the breast as you slide to the armpit. Use enough pressure to tug gently. Repeat this stroke frequently.

Usually, the best technique is to build anticipation by sliding now to the arms or abdomen, and stroking these, returning frequently to the breasts. Conclude breast massage with gentle, local strokes, using fingers, tongue, or lips. Culminate with strokes to the nipples.

HANDS, ARMS, AND FEET

It has been said that the entire female body is an erogenous zone, and that's true to this degree: Although most men would find it pleasant to have their hands and feet caressed, few would find it erotic. Yet, many women do.

A simple finger stroke along the backs of the hands, then the palms, the ankles, tops and bottoms of the feet is all that's necessary. Time and patience are the keys—your partner must know that you're experiencing as much joy as she is.

One effective way to conclude: Using your lips and tongue, begin at the palm of her hand with short, shingled tongue-lapping. Linger there before progressing across the wrist and slowly up the forearm, to the inside of the elbow. Linger there and the chances are good that she'll shudder—the crucial sign of readiness according to the ancient Hindus.

Infants and Children

Warm and protected in the womb, lulled by the rhythmic beat of our mother's heart, nourished without effort and perpetually caressed, we're thrust into the world. For the infant, the great trauma of birth is lost security. Massage can help compensate for this loss.

"Being touched and caressed, being massaged, is food for the infant," says Frederick Leboyer in his book *Loving Hands*. This food is as necessary to the infant as vitamins and minerals, and deprived of it, "babies would rather die. And they often do."

Dr. Ruth Diane Rice, a psychologist specializing in early childhood development, has shown through extensive experiments that when a child is made to feel secure through touch and movement —massage—there is a speeding up of nerve growth, increased cellular activity and endocrine gland function, together with faster weight gain. Those factors can be expected to translate into advanced physical, intellectual, and emotional growth.

All parents should touch and cuddle their babies from birth, and begin half-hour daily routine massages when they're a month or two old. These massages aren't designed to loosen tight muscles, increase circulation or the movement of waste and lymph back to the blood system where they can be excreted by the body. Instead, the massage gives the infant security. Your hands are not the womb, but they're warm and alive. If they're not paradise, they're certainly gentle and strong, and that's why a chronically irritable infant will become serene when it is massaged regularly. Like all of us, an infant is made content when given attention and doted upon.

Another reason infants enjoy massage is that it's simply pleasurable to have one's body caressed—a pleasure perhaps more thoroughly enjoyed by children, who haven't yet absorbed society's mores against the good feelings our bodies can give us. Infants who are often massaged or touched typically grow into adults who feel natural and at ease with their bodies.

The infant taught to equate its body with sin and shame will grow to deny its body and find only illicit, evil, self-destructive pleasure in it, whereas the child who learns to accept naturally and gratefully the pleasures of its body will always have one foot in paradise.

As for you, when you give an infant or child a massage, you'll find it particularly rewarding, often more so than with adults.

That's because children accept what you do for them as their due. When those youngsters reach adolescence, that attitude just might drive you mad, but when an infant stretches out, yawns, smiles, and says in every way he can that you're treating him very nicely, thank you, doing just what he expects of you, there are few experiences so soaringly delightful for a new mother or father.

Finally, your baby will actually learn familiarity with its body through massage. Through the sensation of your hands touching the baby's toes and fingers and limbs, you'll take the first steps toward brain/muscle coordination, and there's evidence that such knowledge early on leads to more rapid intellectual development.

The Setting

If you were your baby, where would you prefer to have a massage? Try to see things from your baby's perspective. Just because you like out-of-doors massage doesn't mean he or she will. The breeze that soothes you might chill your infant. A tiny room that makes you claustrophobic might make the baby feel secure. Silence punctuated by the monotonous ticking of a clock might drive you frantic, but your baby might be soothed immeasurably by it—reminded of your heart's ceaseless pulsing while he or she was in your womb.

Try to think like your infant. Gauge his responses to music, the types that relax him and those that make him irritable. Does the child like the brightness of sunshine or prefer darker, shaded rooms?

The mothers of India sit on the floor with their legs outstretched to form a cradle in which they lay their babies for a massage, and that method has at least three advantages. The infant is embraced on all sides by its mother's warm body; the "cradle" is always instantly available; the distance from "cradle" to floor is minimal, should the infant somehow slip away.

But there are disadvantages, too, especially for Westerners who have grown up with alternatives to hard floors. A cushion can solve the hard floor problem, of course, but many mothers and fathers will find it uncomfortable to keep their legs straight and their bodies upright for the 20 or 30 minutes the massage will take.

I suggest you try this position first for the sake of the intimacy it provides between parent and child, with the help of a thick cushion.

A good alternative is to arrange several throw pillows or sofa cushions in a row on the floor so that you can squat over some of them, half kneeling, half sitting, and lay your baby on the others in front of you. Make sure your knees are protected from the hard floor by pillows or thick carpet.

Expect and prepare for the following:

- Wetting and bowel movements. As your baby completely relaxes, he'll not give a single thought to the mess that might result. Because he really must be naked during a meaningful massage, cover your legs or the pillows first with a waterproof sheet, then a softer one that will feel pleasant against the baby's skin.
- Babies are susceptible to chilling, and they hate it. Make sure the room is warm but not too hot.
- To prevent vomiting, massage the baby while its stomach is empty, but not so close to the next feeding that hunger will distract him from the pleasures of massage.
- Two common reactions babies have to massage are sleep and erections. Both are entirely normal. Neither should interfere with your continuing the massage to completion.

The Baby Massage

From the day your baby is born, you should touch its body for other than the required reasons such as feeding and bathing. It has always surprised me that some men can spend half the night scratching the belly of their German shepherd, yet feel thoroughly ill at ease patting the buttocks of their new baby. I have even known a few women who cheerfully pet their cats but not their babies. It's not that they lack kindness or parental instinct. It simply never occurs to them that children are no different than animals—and adults—in their need for and appreciation of another's touch. Good touching should include gentle squeezing of your baby's arms and legs, patting and playing with fingers and toes.

By the time your child is a month or two old, the touching can gradually lead into actual massage strokes such as those which follow. Obviously, these strokes should be done very lightly, usually with just the fingers. Move very slowly, but not tentatively; as with all massage, your hands must convey a sense of confidence and security. This message of authority from your hands is one of the most important benefits your baby will derive from massage.

1. *Cross-body Slide.* Your baby is lying on his back, his feet toward you. Your hands should be lightly lubricated.

Place your left hand on your baby's left hip—remember, as the infant faces you, his left hip is on your right. Now slide your hand very slowly diagonally across the tiny body toward the right shoulder. As your hand starts across the chest, put your right hand on the baby's right hip and begin a second diagonal stroke to the infant's left shoulder. (If your hands were inked, you'd be smearing an X across your baby's body.)

Continue these alternating strokes until you complete four repetitions. Make sure to maintain contact with the baby's body all the time.

2. *Foot Stroke and Press.* Slide one hand from the shoulder, where you ended the previous stroke, across the abdomen to the leg and down to the foot. Holding the foot with one hand, use one or two fingers from the opposite hand to stroke the top of the foot from ankle to toes.

Lift the leg so that the bottom of your baby's foot faces you. Place your thumb against the soft, fleshy surface and, using light pressure, massage in a small circle.

Unlike that of an adult's, the bottom of the baby's foot is quite sensitive and will remain so until the bones fuse. Very light pressure will tickle, and firm pressure will hurt. Avoid either extreme.

End the foot massage by simply helping your baby to distinguish each of his toes from the others just as mothers always have through the piggly-wiggly game. Hold the big toe in your fingers and move it gently in a circle, then go on to the next toe and repeat. (Three repetitions.)

3. *Leg Squeeze.* Hold your baby's foot at the heel. With your other hand, beginning at the Achilles tendon just above the heel, squeeze the baby's flesh between your thumb and index finger. Move slightly higher, overlapping the previous stroke, and repeat the squeeze. At the ankle, you'll be able to use only the tips of your fingers, but as you move up the leg, you'll probably need more of your fingers and you might even hold the leg in the palm of your hand. Slide over the back of the knee and continue kneading along the hamstring. Slide to the front of the leg at the groin, and continue the stroke down to the knee.

Lower the foot to the cushion. Slide the massaging hand up to the abdomen and across to the other leg. Repeat the entire leg and foot sequence. (Three repetitions.)

Here's another way to judge how much pressure you should use. Always be conscious of the message your hands are conveying to your baby. They're *not* saying, "Relax this muscle, stretch this joint." A healthy baby has no such physiological problems. Your hands are simply saying, "These are your toes, let me introduce them to you. These are your legs, strong and sturdy. This is your torso—it's a lovely torso."

4. *Belly Shingle.* You might think infants are too young to have favorite massage strokes, but in fact they do, and in my experience the belly shingle is the second most popular among babies. (I'll hold you in suspense regarding which is the favorite.)

Place one hand sideways over the baby's pubic area so that your little finger rests just above the pubic bone. Slide your hand slightly upward over the abdomen and chest, then outward to end the stroke at the shoulder.

Before the first hand leaves the baby's body, start the second hand in motion a little higher than where the first stroke began. The stroke is the same, except that the hand moves outward to the opposite side of the baby's body.

When the strokes become so short that they begin on the chest, reverse the direction downward toward the pubic bone and outward. (Three repetitions.)

5. *Face Massage.* Very rare is the infant who enjoys having his face touched—and many won't tolerate it. Your baby will make it clear to you in no uncertain terms what he or she considers pleasant and what is unacceptable.

Babies seem to like forehead massage. Place your thumbs side by side in the middle of your baby's forehead, and move them slowly outward toward the temples. (Repeat, using the shingling effect until you've covered the entire forehead.)

Some practitioners massage the eyelids, above and beneath the eyes, and even the nose, but I find no benefit at all in these techniques. I would simply conclude face massage to infants with another very natural stroke.

Using the index and second fingers of one hand, trace the line from the end of the lips up along the cheekbone and back to the ear. Use not only the tips of the fingers, but the whole flat surface of the finger in a very light, caressing movement. Repeat with the fingers of the other hand on the opposite side of the infant's face. You might try doing the stroke with both hands at once, but very often babies feel somehow trapped and become irritable when they don't have the sense that they can turn their faces away from the fingers if they should choose to. (Three repetitions.)

6. *Arm Tracing.* Techniques for massaging the arms are precisely the same as those used on the legs and feet. The purpose is to help

the baby to become completely aware of its body, which means that you should spend time on each finger, the palm of the hand, the wrist, the elbow, and shoulder joints.

A very pleasant stroke for many babies is a light one-fingered tracing along the back of the hand and up the arm all the way to the shoulder, then back down on the inside of the arm to the palm of the hand. (Three repetitions.)

7. *Whole-Body Slide.* Lay your baby on his stomach crosswise so that his head is to your left, his feet to your right or vice versa. Make sure that he can breathe freely.

Begin with a whole-body slide. With the hand closest to your baby's head, grasp the neck lightly between your thumb and index finger. Your other hand, lubricated, rests at the base of the neck and shoulders, then slowly glides along the spine, over the buttocks, along the backs of one or both legs, and stops at the bottom of the feet. Reverse the stroke, sliding back to the neck. (Two very slow repetitions.)

8. *The Spine Trace.* The spine trace is another pleasant stroke for infants. It follows naturally from the whole-body stroke. Using the thumb and index finger that have lingered at your baby's neck, gently trace the little "valleys" on each side of the spine all the way to the sacrum. While your other hand maintains contact at the baby's buttocks, return the first hand through the air to the neck and repeat the spine trace. (Three repetitions.)

9. *The Buttocks Slide.* The *favorite* stroke of most babies is having their buttocks massaged. As an introductory stroke, use a whole-hand slide from the backs of both thighs up over the entire buttocks, then outward over the hip and return to the upper thighs. (Repeat this relaxing stroke as long as it seems appropriate.)

The baby's buttocks can be gently kneaded, either with thumb and fingers or with two hands pressing the entire buttocks gently together. Experiment to discover the strokes that most delight your baby.

10. *The Buttocks Pat.* For me, the best way to end the massage (and incidentally to put a baby to sleep) is a gentle buttocks patting, using the four fingers of one hand. I don't know why it's so effective—perhaps because it reminds the baby of the rhythmic thumping of the heart against its body while it was in the womb. At any rate, it's the best way I know to put a child to sleep quickly. (Three repetitions.)

At what age should you stop massaging your child? When he himself decides he's too old for it. And the sad fact is that such a day will arrive long before you expect it to.

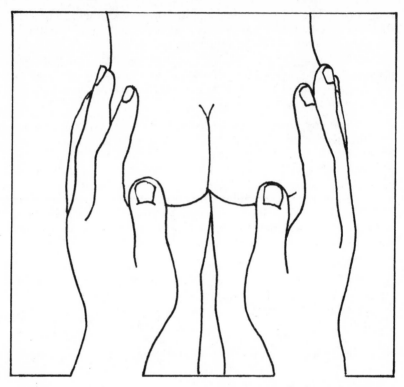

Grandmas and grandpas seem to turn instinctively to gentle buttocks strokes to settle restless infants—or perhaps it's the result of their experience. It's usually much more quick and effective than the jiggling and rocking that younger parents may resort to.

The Aged, Invalid, and Obese

This section is concerned with those whose age, weight, or physical status is a handicap serious enough to warrant special consideration when you give them a massage.

THE AGED

As we grow older, most of us undergo clear-cut physiological changes. I say *most* because research during the last decade has shown that a great many people fail to age "normally"—several measurable functions in their bodies maintain a higher level of efficiency than that of others.

Although part of the explanation for this prolonged youthfulness is certainly genetic, there's no longer any doubt that exercise also plays a major role. I'm going to discuss this in some detail here for a pertinent reason: Among both the elderly and the invalid, massage might be the only form of exercise they get. It's *passive* exercise, not active, and it isn't as good as active, but it's a great deal better than no exercise at all.

The aging process is usually revealed in the following unpleasant physical changes:

- Accumulation of fat.
- Lowering of basal metabolic rates.
- Loss of muscle strength and endurance.
- Reduction in motor fitness—balance, flexibility, agility, and reaction time.
- Reduction in work capacity and associated oxygen intake capacity during attempts at hard work.
- Reduction in respiratory reserves (breath holding and ventilatory capacity).
- Increase in ligamentous injuries and dislocation strains in shoulders, knees, spine, and inguinal region.
- Increase in circulatory problems, blood cholesterol, and blood pressure.
- Decrease in resiliency and suppleness of arteries.
- Progressive bone loss, or osteoporosis, which leads to a weakened and brittle skeletal system.

Massage duplicates many of the benefits of active exercise. Although its effect on fat accumulation is minimal, vigorous, regular massage probably maintains a more active basal metabolic rate, prevents excessive loss in muscle strength and oxygen utilization by increasing circulation. It probably does *not* affect the fitness of the cardiorespiratory system so vital to longevity, but it will help to prevent those common complaints of ligamentous injuries—aches and pains—that plague the elderly. And of course it contributes to keeping the arteries resilient and supple.

In summary, active exercises are preferable, but when your elderly friend simply can't get the exercise he or she should, the next best thing is vigorous, daily whole-body massage.

The Skin. If your friend is elderly, his or her skin is probably dry and perhaps flaky. This is the natural result of decreasingly efficient oil-secreting glands and a reduced level of physical activity, which pulls and tugs the skin, keeping it elastic. What's more, the elderly often shortchange themselves nutritionally. Dry, scaly, and unhealthy skin is one of the first signs of nutritional deficiency.

That means that a lubricating ointment or lotion is essential when you massage an elderly person. Otherwise, a vigorous massage can cause the skin to crack and bleed, or produce an abrasion —a skin burn.

The proper lubricant will not only help you to slide your hands over your friend's body without causing friction, but will enhance skin health, restoring to it essential oil and nutrients. Most lotions rich in lanolin are good. So are coconut, olive, sunflower, and wheat germ oils. These products restore to the skin moisture and nutrients that are quickly absorbed, are natural, and closely resemble the body's own oils.

Vitamins A and E are probably the most important to skin health, and when massaging older men and women I often squeeze two capsules of each of these—10,000 I.U. vitamin A, 400 I.U. vitamin E per capsule—into 4 ounces of oil.

In general, the lotion should contain no irritants. Wintergreen, eucalyptus, and similar heat-producing substances should not be used, nor should acidic substances such as lemon juice and vinegar.

If, during the massage, you've worked the lubricant into the skin sufficiently, it isn't necessary to remove the residue. If, to prevent stains on clothing, you must remove it, avoid using alcohol, which dries the skin. A very mild soap and water solution will do.

Techniques. When you massage an aged or invalid friend, the difference in technique isn't with the strokes—you'll use the same ones you've already learned—but in the method of applying them. In general, the strokes should be lighter than usual. That's especially true of the sliding strokes, which might easily irritate sensitive skin.

When deeper massage is needed, mild compression works well. Use the flat part of your hands and fingers rather than knuckles and fingertips to disperse the pressure over large areas.

Most authorities think that massage for the elderly should be shorter in duration than that for younger people—20 minutes to an hour at the longest. The irony is that older people stand to gain even more from massage than healthy younger people, but the effects cannot be achieved unless you invest time. Particularly when it comes to breaking down fibrous growth and loosening connective tissue to help relieve the stiffness and limited reach of movement so common among the elderly, time and painstaking effort are the key. That means shorter but more frequent massages.

THE INVALID

If your friend is under a doctor's care for illness or injury, get medical approval before giving massage. Your friend's physician will probably be pleased to know that you're willing and able to give massage. Sometimes it can be a real help in promoting healing, even of broken bones and torn muscles, if you know precisely what to do and how to do it. If the doctor knows you're really interested in helping, he or she probably will be glad to take the time to explain what you should and *should not* do.

At other times, the doctor might rule out massage for any number of reasons, including those discussed in Chapter Two. If you keep in mind that massage affects the entire body in some profound ways, it's easy to understand how it could have negative effects under certain conditions. Just one example: Bacteria trapped in a cluster of lymph nodes where they are slowly being destroyed can be spread into the bloodstream through a vigorous massage.

The primary goal in massaging most invalids is to duplicate to some degree the healthy functioning of limbs and muscle groups. Under the guidance of a physician only, limbs that cannot be exercised in the normal way should be "passively exercised"— moved by you through a normal range of function. A doctor can prescribe the number of repetitions for each movement, but the effectiveness is not so much in the number as in the variety. Each muscle and joint that can't be exercised by the invalid should be moved through its full function range. This not only keeps mineral deposits from accumulating in the joints, but it twists and stretches the muscles as normal use would require, helping to maintain tone and suppleness.

THE OBESE

Despite mass advertising to the contrary, you can't sweat fat away with rubberized suits, drink it away with special preparations, or rub it away with magic belts. And you can't massage it away. Fat is stored energy. It comes from high-calorie foods and it's used up through ordinary metabolism and physical activity.

There are no shortcuts. There is no amount of money you can pay to some medical wizard to eliminate fat. That means that you must either reduce your intake of high-calorie foods below the number you burn each day, thereby drawing on the reservoir stored in your body, or you must increase your physical activity sufficiently to require more calories than you eat. The ideal approach is to do both.

Massage won't help eliminate calories—not directly. It *can* contribute in two ways, however. First, studies have shown that overweight people tend to ignore their bodies and do not have an accurate image of their appearance. *Massage focuses their attention on their bodies,* reinforcing the pleasure that can be derived from them. Obviously, someone who is body-conscious is more likely to stick to a diet and exercise program than is someone who can ignore his body.

Most overweight people fail to exercise. Their muscles grow short and stiff, and with the first day of new activity aches and pains are the dubious reward. Both before and after those beginning attempts at activity, stimulating massage can be the key to continuing enthusiasm by preventing or eliminating those aches and pains.

The massage strokes for the obese are the same as those you've already learned, although you'll need to be creative in adapting them, especially to the bodies of very obese people. For example, thumb and index finger kneading of the back will prove useless to someone significantly overweight, but the same effect on underlying muscle can be obtained by using two hands, one moving clockwise, the other counterclockwise, and squeezing and stretching the flesh between them.

Kneading, striking, and compression strokes are most effective in reaching the muscle beneath the layers of excessive fat. Don't make the mistake—common to many beginners—of assuming that fat has no nerve endings. A karate chop to the abdomen meant to stimulate the underlying muscles is just not good technique, regardless of how kind the intent. Your obese friend will no more appreciate being poked, jabbed, pinched, and slapped than you will, for he or she is just as sensitive to pain as you are.

Ordinarily, you can use more pressure than on someone weighing less without causing your friend discomfort. Use hands instead of fingers, your forearm instead of hands. Try using your elbow instead of your thumb when localized treatment is called for.

Always use a positive approach: "You have wonderful muscle tone—I can *feel* it." "Your basic body structure is really impressive."

A little psychology can go a long way in motivating your obese friend toward losing weight.

PART III
FINGER PRESSURE
MASSAGE FOR PAIN RELIEF

CHAPTER SEVEN

THE FUNDAMENTALS OF FINGER PRESSURE MASSAGE

From the beginning, massage was used for healing.

The world's first medical textbook, written in 4000 B.C., was also as detailed a guide to massage as had ever been written. *The Yellow Emperor's Classic of Internal Medicine,* published in China, described some of the strokes which the Greeks later perfected and which are now part of classical massage. But the overwhelming emphasis in *The Yellow Emperor's Classic* is on an entirely different technique based not on whole-body strokes but on localized finger pressure.

For thousands of years before finger pressure techniques were described in writing, Chinese physicians had used and perfected finger pressure as the primary Oriental healing art. The specific form of finger pressure practiced by the Chinese (there are a number of others as you'll see) is known today by its Japanese name— *shiatsu.*

Another type of finger pressure massage is *pressure point.* In 1893, a fellow named Cornelius found himself bedridden for several months with a severe streptococcal infection. Virtually all the joints of his body were swollen and painful, and there was no sign of improvement until one of the medical officers assigned to give Cornelius daily massages began to use an unusual technique. Cornelius wrote, "He palpated the area and where he found pain, he dwelled longer than elsewhere."

Cornelius later pressed the painful areas himself and instructed his masseur to do the same. He reported:

The success was astonishing. Swelling as well as pain disappeared in a very short time and while previously I had not experienced the least improvement . . . after four weeks of this kind of massage I was free of swelling and discomfort and was able to return to duty, apparently completely recovered and feeling strong and healthy . . .

Cornelius had found that firm pressure on a sensitive spot could relieve pain, either by anesthetizing the nerves, forcing a muscle in spasm to relax, or both. The result was a spate of practitioners using finger pressure techniques similar in many ways to those of Cornelius, among them heartspann (heart-tone), palpatory massage, contact massage, and zone therapy.

One of the most recent finger pressure techniques is myotherapy. In November 1980, the well-known physical fitness expert Bonnie Prudden described in *McCall's* magazine what an editor apparently headlined "A revolutionary technique to stop muscular pain." Myotherapy is certainly effective—but much of myotherapy is as old as *The Yellow Emperor of China.*

For many modern practitioners, it has a significant advantage over the ancient pressure point therapy—which Prudden calls *trigger points;* it sidesteps philosophy and theory in favor of practice. Prudden goes directly to the most sensitive spot in a painful muscle. These trigger points develop all through life—even the birth process can produce the first batch of trigger points, she says.

"A trigger point lies quietly in a muscle until the emotional climate is right, and then it 'fires,' " she states. That trigger point causes the muscle to go into spasm. The spasm causes pain—and the pain leads to greater spasm. Until the muscle is somehow relaxed, it continues its painful shortening and contraction. That's nature's way of keeping you from using the muscle while it's trying to heal, but it's another example of the body overreacting, as it does in allergies, for example—the body's "cure" is worse than the ailment.

Prudden's technique is to apply up to 35 pounds of pressure directly to the trigger point, holding it for about 7 seconds, except on the face and head, where 4 or 5 seconds is sufficient. As the pressure is relaxed, the pain disappears, sometimes temporarily and often for good.

In the following chapters, you'll learn to use some of the major finger pressure techniques. I will not tell you that by mastering them you will be capable of bestowing the gift of healing—only God and the body can heal. But I will promise you this: Through these techniques you will be able to relieve many kinds of pain, from minor aches to crippling spasms. And that is a very worthwhile gift to have.

When to Use Finger Pressure Massage

Today finger pressure is always used for a specific job. Here are some of the reasons to choose finger pressure:

- It relieves pain caused directly or indirectly by muscle spasm. If that seems of minor importance, keep in mind that most *functional* pain—that which results from the way we use or misuse our bodies rather than from organic disease or deterioration—originates in our muscles. The relief might be temporary, or it might be permanent.
- The relief of pain from finger pressure massage helps to reduce overall body tension, with the obvious results: improved emotional health, sleeping habits, and sense of well-being. But it also reduces the likelihood of another muscle, remote from the original site, going into spasm because of the excessive tension on it.
- Depending on the cause of the muscle spasm (or splinting or cramping), finger pressure massage might actually effect a cure.

Our primary focus will be on functional ailments, the everyday aches, pains, spasms, and strains that don't quite cripple us but leave us with stiff necks, aching backs, arms we can't lift above our shoulders, thighs and feet that make us limp. Years of poor posture could have caused that chronic, nagging pain. Or the culprit might have been a pair of shoes that didn't fit properly. Every step might have subtly twisted your foot out of alignment, placing continuous stress on muscles not only in your legs but also the lower back. Finally, those muscles might have reacted by going into a protective spasm.

Potential causes of functional pain involving the muscles could fill a book. Any trauma could easily create an abnormal alignment of muscle and bone that, even decades later, as nerves are pinched or muscles stretched, might lead to pain. A mishap on a bicycle, an auto accident, a strain while lifting a heavy object, a sudden twist of the neck—these are some of the more common muscle "insults" or abuses that can lead to muscle spasms and acute or chronic pain.

That's the pain you'll learn to relieve in the following sections.

When Not to Use Finger Pressure

Finger pressure massage can often spare your friend an unnecessary and expensive trip to the doctor. Rarely, it can do even more —although a physician prescribes drugs and perhaps surgery, some conditions can be cured by nothing more elaborate than your thumbs. That's not common, granted, but such cases do occur.

Yet, I don't advocate using *any* finger pressure massage as an exclusive treatment for serious organic illness. Wise men have long recognized that only a fool puts all his eggs in one basket, and although some practitioners have claimed many successes in curing stomach pain, a persistent sufferer would be wise to have his or her medical doctor rule out ulcers, cancer, and other serious possibilities before deciding on finger pressure massage alone.

The same point holds for symptoms that indicate any potentially serious illness.

Generally a good rule of thumb regarding pain of unknown cause is this: If the pain is severe and/or seems to be related to a vital organ, seek a medical diagnosis immediately. If the pain is moderate and is skeletal/muscular in nature (that includes arthritic pain), finger pressure is likely to be dramatically beneficial. If so, good to excellent results should occur immediately.

If after three or four applications several hours apart you see no positive results, it's time to consider medical help.

Finally:

- Don't use finger pressure massage on a mole, wart, varicose vein, swelling, inflammation, or severe scar that isn't fully healed.
- Don't use it on the abdomen of a pregnant woman or upon the breasts of any woman.
- Don't use it on fractured bones, torn ligaments, burns, cuts, or other trauma injuries. In a nutshell, use common sense.

CHAPTER EIGHT

TECHNIQUES IN FINGER PRESSURE MASSAGE

The Pressure Points

Almost all finger pressure massage techniques, whether their goal is simply to relieve functional pain of muscular origin or to perform virtual miracles of visceral healing, have something in common: They all use *pressure points*.

HOW THEY WORK

When we offer explanations about *how* pressure point massage works, we're discussing theory, as I said earlier, not fact. Granted, these theories have been offered by experts in the field, and that expertise warrants serious consideration of their ideas. Even the fact that the experts disagree in their theories doesn't necessarily disprove any of them—the relief of pain might result from a symphony of factors rather than a single one.

Here's what we *know:*

Pain so severe that it might be crippling, and never correctly diagnosed in spite of a battery of highly sophisticated medical tests, can often be relieved in a matter of minutes through pressure at the proper muscle or tendon locations. We *know* that finger pressure works to relieve pain. We *believe* that it does so by causing a muscle in spasm to relax.

The question is why the muscle relaxes. One theory is that the

body sends endorphins to the area. These are morphine-like substances, but many times more powerful, produced naturally in the
body to block pain signals throughout the body. But pain, remember, is indispensable to our survival—it gets our hands out of the
fire, tells us we've been in the sun too long. The body doesn't
protect us from what it considers "good" pain.

The muscle spasm is the body's way of protecting itself from
further injury. If the pain were eased, we might stress the muscle
again and risk further damage. So, the endorphins are not forthcoming in this case.

When finger pressure is applied, however, having nothing to do
with the original threat to the muscle, the body theoretically re-
leases endorphins to deal with that particular trauma.

A second theory is that pressure at the precise point where the
seat of the spasm exists temporarily cuts off circulation, thereby
depriving the tissue of oxygen. Oxygen-starved tissue cannot
function. Figuratively speaking, the muscle slips into "unconsciousness," such as you and I would if we were deprived of oxygen. The injured muscle relaxes, and when it begins functioning
again, it's no longer painful.

Finally, the spasm relaxation phenomenon might be similar to
the results produced by stretch exercise. If you sit on the floor
with your legs outstretched and try to touch your forehead to your
knees, you might find it difficult. If you're typical, you'll feel the
tightness in your back and hamstring muscles. But if you hold for
a moment the most extreme position you can tolerate, you'll notice
that what was at first a very uncomfortable position suddenly feels
quite normal. The muscle "gives up," stretches, and relaxes, and
you can lower your head several more inches toward your knees.

It might be that putting pressure on a muscle spasm actually
does stretch the tissue in a very limited area—or at least produces
the same effect as stretching. The result, at any rate, appears to
be the same.

One of the most important benefits of finger pressure massage
is the way it relieves *referred pain*. Most of us have undergone
physical examinations during which the doctor slugged our kneecap with a rubber mallet, causing our foot to rise involuntarily.
That's known as the knee jerk reaction. We never give it a thought
—in fact, that very expression (knee jerk reaction) has come to
mean thoughtless robotlike behavior.

If we *did* stop to think about it, we might find it quite amazing
that a blow to the knee can cause a leg muscle to go into spasm.

According to legend, that sort of referred response was first recognized more than 5000 years ago when, in the midst of battle, an

arrow pierced the leg of a Chinese soldier. He was a very level-headed soldier indeed, for, despite the pain in his leg and the battle raging around him, he took time to ponder the fact that the instant the arrow pierced his leg his stomachache disappeared!

A comrade made a similar discovery: A wound of the hand relieved him of the migraines he'd suffered all his life. These chance occurrences are said to have led to the discovery of acupuncture.

I mention this simply to illustrate that humankind has recognized for a very long time that seemingly unexplainable pain in one part of the body can be referred from muscle tension or spasm elsewhere. There are at least three ways that this can happen:

• The muscle spasm can involve a nerve branch to the distant site where this pain seems to be occurring. An example: the patient who has had his leg amputated, yet complains of severe pain in the foot he no longer possesses. The nerve trunk that once served the foot and now ends at the stump continues to send pain messages back to the brain.

• Blood circulation to the painful site might be reduced by the muscle spasm elsewhere, and that deprivation can cause pain.

• A muscle spasm in one area can tug violently on bones, tendons, and ligaments, causing a chain-reaction tension and producing stress and pain in weaker muscles elsewhere.

WHERE THEY ARE

The most common question I'm asked concerning finger pressure massage (especially by those with some knowledge of the subject) is: "Are the pressure points the same as the tsubos of shiatsu and Bonnie Prudden's trigger points, and the zones in connective tissue massage and reflexology?"

The answer is—sometimes.

Some pressure points can be found at or near the Oriental tsubos. Others will coincide with trigger points and others with reflex zones.

Although many practitioners can point to their charts to show exactly where pressure points are located, the fact is that no one can tell you *precisely* where a given pressure point is located on a particular individual. Besides, it's not necessary. Instead, in the following sections, I'll illustrate with drawings the general areas likely to be responsible for local and referred pain, but within that general area, you yourself will *search* for the pressure points involved.

It's a simple process, actually, for whenever a pressure point is responsible for pain—either local or referred—it's highly sensitive to pressure. By *searching* the area indicated in the illustrations, you'll identify the pressure points involved—your friend will let you know when you've found the painful spots. Through this method, you'll avoid the need to labor over complex road maps of the body, and concentrate on the treatment itself.

Keep in mind that the pain you're treating will probably be related to more than one pressure point and that, even if you treat the point most directly responsible, you could fail to relieve the pain—or, at best, relieve it only temporarily—if you ignore the other points.

Pressure points often behave sympathetically; when one becomes severely irritated, surrounding points also become sensitive and contribute to the overall pain. So, don't be content to find the point primarily responsible for your friend's complaint, but check out all the points potentially related to the painful area.

To find the precise location of the pressure points, use your fingertip, thumb, or knuckle (depending on the thickness of the muscle involved), and press *firmly* on that part of your friend's body that corresponds with the dark circle in the shaded area of the applicable illustration. The pressure should be obvious, but not really painful unless that point needs treatment. If your friend feels no unusual pain after a few seconds, relax the pressure, move your finger slightly, and repeat, continuing until you've covered every part of the shaded area.

At some point, your friend will announce a twinge of unusually sharp pain as you discover the sensitive pressure point. You might want to mark that spot with a felt-tipped pen or a dab of lipstick while you continue to search for remaining sensitive pressure points. Then, treat them one by one, beginning with the primary point—the one obviously most sensitive.

Treatment Techniques

Finger pressure massage, obviously, is applied with your fingers, usually the thumbs, but you can use any finger that's strong enough to maintain real pressure. If you're treating muscles of the arms or lower legs, you might use your knuckles and, for the large muscles of the back, buttocks, and thighs, your elbow can be the perfect tool for finger pressure—even though it's not a finger.

The "pressure" in finger pressure is generally static—your finger doesn't slide over your friend's skin but remains in the same place of moves *with* the skin for just an inch or less. So, unlike classical massage, no oils, lotions, or powders should be used in finger pressure.

The technique you use will depend to a great extent on the part of the body you're treating, just as they do in classical massage. In general, finger pressure should be applied to the *precise* point of sensitivity with enough pressure to cause pain—"to make you wince," as one authority says—but not *intolerable* pain. The pressure should be held for 7 to 10 seconds, but there is an even better criterion for judging when the pressure has been held long enough: Ask your friend to tell you when the sharp pain caused by the finger pressure vanishes.

The key to firm pressure without straining yourself is to use your weight, not your strength. Learn to lock your fingers firmly, then lean into them. Your fingernails should be cut short and filed smooth.

Finger pressure massage for any single muscle pain should be brief. Treating the primary pressure point as well as satellites might take as little as a minute or as much as five minutes, but rarely more. You can do more harm than good by continuing to press points that have already relaxed.

Some people need more specific guidelines regarding the amount of pressure to use. Where feasible, I'll offer my preference, in terms of pounds of pressure, which will vary from 5 to 35 pounds. If it's easier for you to work with this kind of information than to rely on your own instinct and sensitivity, practice recognizing how much pressure 5 pounds to 35 pounds is by using your bathroom scale. Try to determine how much muscular effort goes into each individual 5 pounds. (The one thing you simply can't do while giving massage is to stop for a "scale break" so that you can get the pressure just right.)

Have your friend lie either on the floor or on a table—not a bed, because that will require you to bend over too far, putting a strain on your back muscles. (Then *you'll* be the one needing massage.)

After your friend receives finger pressure massage, he or she should relax for a few minutes before moving or exercising the treated area. During that time, you might want to give a full-body general massage or a casual back rub.

CHAPTER NINE

GIVING A FINGER PRESSURE MASSAGE

Head, Neck, and Shoulders

Headaches, stiff necks and aching tension in the upper back and shoulder muscles share this distinction: 80 to 90 percent of the time, they arise from *involuntary muscle tension*. And they can often be relieved through the proper finger pressure massage.

Headaches

I've yet to meet a person who has never suffered a headache, and more than 12 million of us have had the worst kind—migraine. The pain of a migraine is so severe that it can cause vomiting, screaming, and even unconsciousness. Sufferers have been known to bang their heads against solid objects, stick them in freezers and in ovens to seek relief.

Headaches were diagnosed thousands of years ago. In some cultures, the treatment of choice was to drill a hole through the skull so that the evil spirits causing the pain could escape. Today, the usual treatment is drugs, but they're not always effective, because a given headache might not be caused by the problem a particular drug is designed to treat.

Finger pressure massage can be a very effective therapy for headache pain but, like drugs, its effectiveness depends on the cause of the headache.

One reason it has taken humankind so long to come up with effective treatments for so common an ailment is that we assumed that pain in our heads was caused by an ailment right there where it hurt. But, as one authority, J. Calvin Davis, M.D., has pointed out, head pain might well be associated with "pathological processes of the eyes, ears, teeth, nerves, vascular system, and other parts of the body."

A headache can be caused by arthritis in the neck, heart disease, drugs (both legal and illegal), food allergies, infections—any number of organic ailments anywhere in the body. In fact, a report in the *Journal of the American Medical Association* documented a case of recurrent headache related to fever blisters and chancre sores of the lips, mouth, and nose.

Yet, according to Arnold P. Friedman, M.D., of Columbia University, writing in *Postgraduate Medicine* (Vol. 53, No. 6), "chronic recurrent headache can be divided into two main diagnostic categories . . . these are vascular headaches of the migraine type and muscle-contraction (tension) headache."

Now, here's the important point: Dr. Friedman says, in *85 to 90 percent* of cases of chronic recurrent headache, the attack is vascular headache of the migraine type or of the *muscular-contraction* type, or a combination of these.

Muscle-contraction headaches can *always* be helped by proper finger pressure massage, and those vascular headaches that are related to muscle contraction—in which tight muscles constrict the blood vessels, either limiting blood supply or causing congestion or both—can also be treated effectively by finger pressure massage.

Headaches of emotional origin can also be treated by massage, a combination of finger pressure and classical techniques designed to relax muscles as a prelude to psychological relaxation.

And finger pressure massage can ease sinus congestion, together with the headaches caused by that condition. In fact, some authorities believe that massage can control or eliminate all but about 5 percent of headaches.

Obviously, that 5 percent can be a warning of serious illness— meningitis, a tumor, or some other life-threatening condition. If massage doesn't ease your friend's headache promptly, be sure that he or she sees a doctor for an accurate diagnosis.

On the illustrations accompanying these chapters on finger pressure massage, the dotted areas indicate where you will find pressure points, and the dark circles show more precisely where they're *usually* found. The accompanying text will explain how many points exist in each dotted area—but keep in mind that not all of the points will necessarily be sensitive. If they are not, *don't* treat them, or you might cause the muscles to contract protectively and create a problem where none existed previously. You *should*, however, search the entire shaded area, even if you've already found one sensitive pressure point. It's possible that more than one—or perhaps each—point in the area is sensitive and should be treated.

Pressure Areas of the Face

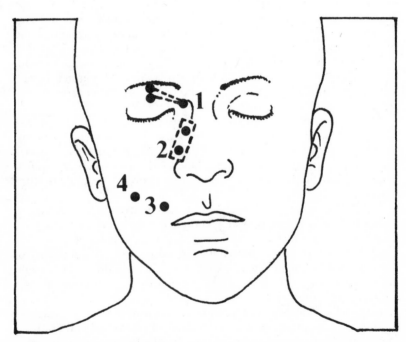

Facial areas 1, 2, 3, and 4. The easiest way to find area 4 is to have your friend open her mouth wide and begin searching below the cheekbone on the outer edge of the jaw muscle. This is a sensitive point, and your friend will let you know when you've found it.

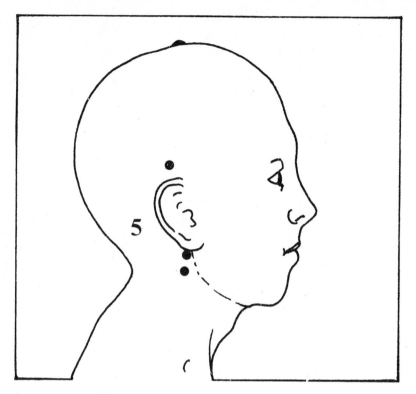

Face area 5.

Area 1. There are five major pressure point areas in the face. The *first* includes the *eye points,* of which there are three. One is where the eyebrow joins the bridge of the nose. Press up against the underside of the eyebrow bone to find this point.

The second is on the underside of the eyebrow at the midpoint above the eye.

The third is in that same area, but farther back in the eye socket. Rest your fingernail against the second point and press the tip of your finger forward until it touches (gently) the eyeball—the point is on that bone above the eyeball. Use very little pressure on these last two areas—they are highly sensitive.

Area 2. This area includes the *nasal points,* of which there are two. The first is just below the eye socket beside the nose. The other is between the nostril and cheekbone. About 6 pounds of pressure can be used here, depending on your friend's sensitivity.

Area 3. The *third* is the *mouth point,* above and to the outer edge of the upper lip and just beneath the cheekbone. On some people this point is closer to the nose, on others it is more toward the outside of the face.

Area 4. The *fourth* pressure area in the face is in the *jaw muscle.* Ask your friend to open his or her mouth. At the edge of the muscle, just before it gives way to the hollowness of the cheek, is the pressure point.

Area 5. The *fifth* face area, with three points, is around the *ear.* Point 1 is at the hollow behind the ear, where the ear bone and jawbone meet. Press up toward the ear. The second point is a fraction of an inch below. Press not inward but sideward against the jawbone. Point 3 is directly above point one, 1 to 2 inches above the top of the ear.

Use moderate pressure on points 1 and 2, firm pressure on point 3.

In addition to the face points, another exists in the *center of the skull.* Imagine a line extending from the tip of the nose upward between the eyes toward the forehead and around the head—and another line extending from ear to ear. Where they intersect is the pressure point. To find the precise location, search from forehead to back of skull rather than from ear to ear. You can use a good deal of pressure on this point, but do not stimulate this area at all in young children, whose cranial bones are not yet fully fused.

Pressure Areas of the Neck

One of the fascinating things you're going to discover as you use finger pressure massage to relieve your friend's headache is that, with few exceptions (such as sinus, ear, and jaw muscle-related headaches), the problem causing the pain isn't in the head at all but in the neck. That's one reason why learning finger pressure massage of the neck is so valuable.

Another is that the neck not only causes the head pain, but has its own assortment of aches and pains to suffer. Fall asleep at night with your head in a slightly unusual position and there's every chance you'll wake up in the morning with what our grand-parents call a "crook in the neck." Turn your head suddenly, and there it is again, a pain so severe that the next time you turn your head, you'll have to turn your whole body as well.

Sit with your head bent over a book for an hour or two and you'll stand tall only by resisting the stiffness.

Those problems don't occur among the young, usually, and there's good reason: As we grow older, our necks are the first to tell us the news. Many delicate bones make up the thin spinal column of our necks. If even small amounts of calcium deposits and uric acid crystals clutter the spaces between these bones, the creaking and cracking sounds of middle-aged necks announce that the bones are no longer gliding across each other smoothly.

But it's not the debris between moving bones that causes most pain. It's another kind of accumulation, that of tension, and it can cause contraction in the muscles from the base of our skulls down to our buttocks, from our shoulders to our jaws. This tension both exhausts us and gives us headaches—and it can pull those bones more tightly together, causing wear and tear.

Finger pressure massage can relieve that tightness, together with accompanying pain.

Search all the points illustrated and described and press those that are sensitive with 10 to 20 pounds of pressure, whether you're treating headaches, stiff necks, or other neck symptoms.

Area 1. This area (see the illustration on page 114) is located at the base of the skull, spreading out to the midpoint between the center of the neck and each ear.

Pressure point 1 is just above the last vertebra that you can feel, in the indentation just below the skull.

There is another indentation between the first and second ver-tebra—that's pressure point 2.

Slide your finger outward from the vertebrae just below the skull so that the side of your finger is actually tracing the skull bone, and you'll find the *third* and *fourth* pressure points as you reach the slight bulge of the sternocleidomastoid muscle on the side of the neck behind the ear.

These last two points are major culprits in causing or sustaining tension headaches—in fact, if one area only is involved, this will probably be it.

Area 2. If area 1 could be called the headache zone, area 2, which includes the neck aspect of the trapezius muscle, is the overall tension zone. You'll recall that, in discussing classical massage, I explained that the most effective relaxation massage concentrates

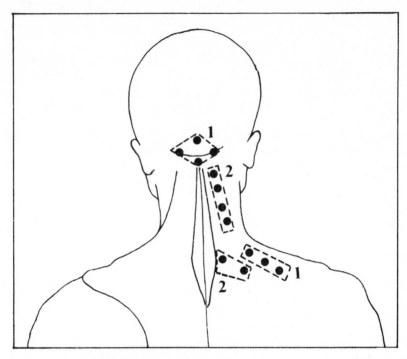

Neck areas 1 and 2. Shoulder areas 1 and 2.

on precisely this muscle, which originates at the skull, flares out to the shoulders, then plunges in a sharp V halfway down the back, connecting along that entire length of the spine. When tension builds, it usually accumulates first in the trapezius.

There are four pressure points in neck area 2, occurring in sets of two, on each side of the spinal column below the scalp. They will tolerate, and appreciate, firm pressure of about 15 pounds.

With practice, you can press one area on each side of the spine simultaneously by grasping the back of your friend's neck between your thumb and forefinger and squeezing. The advantage is that, as both parts of the muscle relax, there is less chance of sympathetic spasm occurring in the nonpressed point.

Area 3. Have your friend turn his or her head to the side and note the muscle that bulges from the ear to the collarbone. This muscle, the sternocleidomastoid, is usually responsible for neck pain and stiffness. If it is allowed to become less flexible, any sudden turn of the head in one direction can stretch the muscle

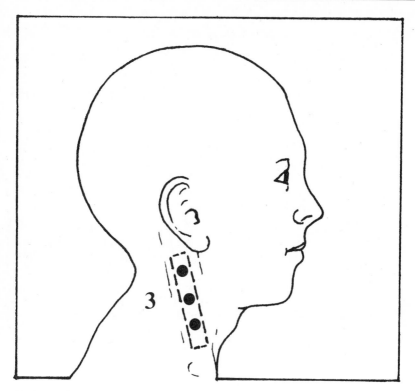

Neck area 3.

on the opposite side of the neck, causing it to contract in a protective cramp.

The sternocleidomastoid harbors three major pressure points. The *first* is at the highest part of the muscle, where it connects to the skull bone. The *second* is approximately even with the chin line of the jaw—if your drew a line from the chin along the jaw, it would point approximately to this pressure point. And the *third* point is approximately at the same level as the highest part of the throat.

These points can be pressed in traditional fashion or, more effective in my opinion, they can be squeezed between thumb and forefinger.

Pressure Areas of the Shoulder

There are *three major pressure areas* of the shoulders, and on them you can use heavy pressure—about 25 pounds. All of them are found in the trapezius, which at first touch might feel almost impenetrable because of the tension.

Area 1. This area is easily found by placing your right hand on your friend's left shoulder as he faces you, your thumb against his neck, and your fingers lying flat on the top of the shoulder. The tips of the fingers will rest across all three pressure points on the back of his shoulder. (See the drawing on page 114 for shoulder areas 1 and 2.)

Area 2. This area is also easy to find because the points here are particularly sensitive in most people. Begin your search near but not on the spine for the *first* large, knotted pressure point. This is a key point and is almost always involved in shoulder tension. If you place your small finger on this point, your index or middle finger will be on or very close to the *second* pressure point.

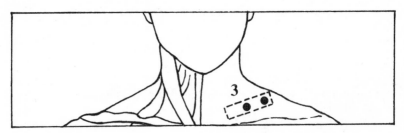

Shoulder area 3 (for shoulder areas 1 and 2, see illustration on page 114).

Area 3. This area is on the front of the shoulder, just above the point where the trapezius connects to the clavicle. Ask your friend to turn his head to the left so that the sternocleidomastoid protrudes on the right side of his neck. Place your index finger against —not on—that muscle, *approximately* an inch above the clavicle, and your remaining fingers will be covering these *two* pressure points. Ask your friend to face forward again before searching for them.

The Back

Years ago doctors thought backache was caused by our upright posture. They said that the vertebrae and discs are forced into abnormal positions when we stand on two legs instead of four. The resulting pressures from sudden movement cause the back problems.

Even today this point of view is quite popular, especially among laypersons—even though there is little evidence to support it. Instead, medical science is becoming more and more convinced that our backs are victims of sedentary living.

Among the many researchers now certain of that is Hans Kraus, M.D., clinical associate professor of physical medicine and rehabilitation at New York University. He has been working with backache sufferers for many years, and is one of the nation's leading authorities on the subject. His conclusion: "We should look at most of the back and neck pain sufferers as persons whose condition is caused by physical inactivity under circumstances which combine lack of exercise with emotional stress and strain."

Studies indicate that more than 80 percent of low back pain is caused by our sedentary life-style. Either our muscles are too weak, or they are too stiff and tense, or they become too short.

Let's take a more careful look at each of the three major causes of backache.

At the first sign of backache, some people make it a point to sit absolutely straight—perfect posture, they call it—every waking moment. It's part of the old-fashioned idea that backache is inevitably related to poor posture.

The fact is, the very muscular rigidity involved in maintaining that "perfect" posture may be the cause of backache. Muscle rigidity can come from remaining in the same position without moving for prolonged periods, with the muscles in a constant state of tension.

"It is often evident," says Dr. Kraus, "that maintaining a fixed position for prolonged periods may cause discomfort—even if that position complies with the ideal postural requirements. Holding muscles rigid will in itself produce stiffness, muscle tension and pain."

Muscle tension can also come from emotional tension—and that in itself may well be the leading cause of backache among most people who have high-pressure jobs. One commercial artist found that he developed a severe backache of several days' duration once a month. He tried new chairs, improved posture—but nothing worked to relieve the pain. Finally, he recognized that backaches always coincided with the days that he was forced to work on a high-pressure deadline account. It was the most taxing part of his schedule, and only his best work was good enough. Once he realized that, he began relaxation exercises combined with finger pressure massage—and the pain vanished.

Says Dr. Kraus, "The initial attack of back pain is frequently precipitated by emotional problems, tension, business strain . . ."

Weak abdominal and back muscles may be the cause of persistent backache. Dr. Kraus and his colleague Dr. Weber have developed a test to determine if muscles are excessively weak. In abbreviated form, it's a simple test you can undertake in a few minutes. Here it is, step-by-step:

1. Lie on your back with hands behind your neck and legs extended. Lift your feet off the floor and hold the position for 10 seconds.
2. Starting in the same position as before, lean forward into a sitting position. Don't keep your back straight, but bend it forward as you rise up. Keep your hands behind your neck.
3. Starting from the same position, but knees bent this time, hands behind your neck, lean forward into the sitting position.
4. Lie on your stomach, a pillow beneath your abdomen. Keep your hands behind your neck. Have a friend hold your feet and hips in place. Raise your head and chest off the floor and hold that position for 10 seconds.
5. In the same starting position, have your friend hold your head and back down. Without bending your knees, lift your feet and legs from the floor. Hold for 10 seconds.
6. Stand erect in bare feet and bend slowly and without straining to see how close you can come to touching your feet. (Although the Kraus-Weber test would have you keep your knees stiff, I advocate that the knees be slightly bent to avoid knee and tendon damage.)

If you find that you can't pass these minimal tests, there's no question but that you have weak or short muscles.

But back problems can also be caused by muscles not in our backs. Many of us have jobs that require more or less continuous sitting for eight hours a day, and our evening activities are often chair-oriented, too. The hip flexors, which attach between the top of the thighbones and the ilium, automatically shorten when you lower your hips to sit down. The hamstring muscles on the back of the thighs and legs shorten when the knees are bent. The result is that these muscles may become permanently short, making it impossible to stand erect and assume a normal relaxed posture because of the pull of these muscles. The back muscles may be overworked and vertebrae can be pulled out of alignment. That's the path to a chronic backache.

The best *treatment* for most back problems is *stretch exercises*. Chapter Fourteen is devoted entirely to stretch exercises, for there's nothing more important that you can do for your body—or your friend's—in harmony with massage to help your muscles stay relaxed and supple.

Stretch exercises will help to keep those massive back muscles from tensing and those trigger points from becoming excessively sensitive. But if your friend is actually suffering back pain, pressure point massage should be the very first thing you do—*after* priority number one, which is to eliminate the possibility of damage to the spine. If your friend is sure that she hasn't injured herself through a fall or other accident, and that the pain is unrelated to the spinal column, *then* you can begin pressure point massage.

Pressure Areas of the Upper Back

You're already familiar with the concept of referred, or reflex, pain, and here on the upper back, you'll find one of the two most common sources of that problem in the entire body. (The second, and most frequent source is pain felt in the lower back and referred from the buttocks, which we'll talk about later.)

Pressure points in the upper back *always* become sensitive when upper back muscles are tight or in spasm, but that doesn't necessarily mean that the back muscles are relaying pain messages to your brain. Instead, these incredibly strong muscles might be quite capable of handling the stress of spontaneous spasms. Without your being at all aware of it, they might continue to grow tighter and shorter for years, pulling skeletal structures to which they're attached out of line, causing postural defects. Eventually, all this leads to stress on weaker muscles—and when the pain finally begins, it might be in them. Usually, your *back* literally becomes a pain in the *neck*.

If pressure points in the neck and shoulders fail to relieve neck pain, the origin of the problem is almost certainly the upper back muscles.

Area 1. While your friend is lying on her abdomen, kneel at her head and rest the *heel* of your right hand on the edge of her left shoulder, with your fingers pointing toward her right hip. The balls of your fingers will be resting on the first of *two pressure points* in area 1. Search it out and compress it. This is the deltoid muscle and, like most back muscles, it will require a great deal of pressure to give results—30 pounds or more, depending on your friend's ability to tolerate pain.

Search for the second point along a straight line from where your fingertips are and directly toward the spine. The point is at the spot where the deltoid and trapezius meet. (Actually, a third muscle, the infraspinatus, also intersects at this point, so pressure here actually affects three major muscles.)

Area 2. There are *three* primary pressure points here, beginning at the armpit level about halfway between the two pressure points in area 1 and extending 3 or 4 inches toward the hip and parallel with the spine.

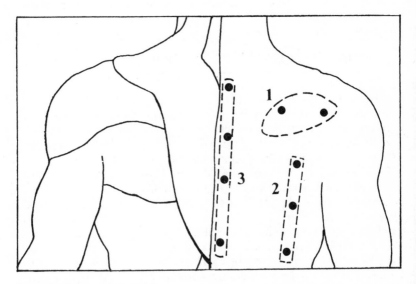

Upper back areas 1, 2, and 3.

Area 3. All four pressure points in area 3 are located in the trapezius, in the tiny valley next to—but not on—the spine. Begin searching just below the point on the lower neck where the firmness of the lumbodorsal fascia gives way to the softer muscle tissue, and continue to where the tissue loses its resiliency as the firmer fascia flares outward again (about halfway to the waist). Although there are *four major pressure points* in area 3, you might find minor ones that are also sensitive and need treatment.

Pressure Areas of the Lower Back

Here's the most common site of back pain, and it's the first place you should search for spasm pressure points when your friend complains of pain in this area. Chances are, three minutes of treatment here will bring relief so dramatic it will seem almost miraculous.

If lower back pain eases but doesn't disappear when you treat pressure points in this region, the irritation is almost certainly secondary to that of primary spasms in the gluteal muscles (see the next section).

Area 1. This area of the lower back contains just one pressure point, and its easy to find. It's on the rise of muscle next to the

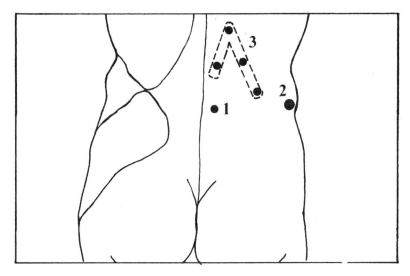

Lower back areas 1, 2, and 3.

spine, and along the beltline. Sometimes you might find additional sensitive spots along the beltline, but this is the major point.

Area 2. This area is on the outer edge of the beltline, above the hipbone, in the external oblique muscle. Some people are ticklish at this spot, but they won't laugh if you press hard enough—15 pounds of steady pressure.

Area 3. This area contains four pressure points. Lay the heel of your right hand on the right side of your friend's back at her beltline, midway between areas 1 and 2. Your thumbs should be extended toward area 1, your fingers together and pointing toward your friend's neck. With your hand in that position, your fingers are lying across three of the four pressure points in area 3. They're on the line where the latissimus dorsi connects to the lumbodorsal fascia, and you can feel the soft muscle give way to the tougher tendon. Search carefully for each of these points, particularly the middle one, and apply strong pressure to each.

The fourth point in area 3 is located almost directly above area 1. It forms the apex of a triangle composed of the four points in area 3. The easiest way to locate it is to search upward from area 1 beside the spine. You'll find it an inch or two above the lower point.

The Buttocks

Two years ago, while vacuuming the family room, my wife Alice sank to her knees, lay back on the carpet, and cried. The bent-over position she'd assumed while vacuuming had triggered excruciating pain in her lower back.

Eight years earlier the same thing had happened. My training in those days was primarily in nutrition, exercise physiology, and classical massage, and I'd just begun studying finger pressure massage. I'd applied pressure to the major points of Alice's lower back, but she'd felt only slight, temporary relief.

Two days later, she still could hardly get out of bed, so I telephoned the doctor and got a prescription. The name of the drug escapes me now (that was 10 years ago), but I recall researching its potential side effects in *Physicians' Desk Reference*. The drug included steroids, and the possible side effects were many, including bone softening, and kidney and liver damage. Alice had no choice—the pain was unbearable—so she took the drug. After two days, the pain eased sufficiently for her to discontinue using it.

When the back pain recurred two years ago, she was again vacuuming the family room. But this time, I knew a great deal about finger pressure massage, having used it on scores of friends, acquaintances, and relatives. I helped Alice to roll over onto her stomach, lifted her arms gently above her head, then applied pressure to all the lower back points discussed in the previous section. When relief was only minimal, I knew for certain that the back pain *was being referred from a muscle spasm in the gluteals, or buttocks*. In less than a minute, I'd discovered the exact primary pressure point, applied 10 seconds of firm force, and helped my relieved—and astonished—wife to her feet.

Yes, it was painful for the first few seconds as I pressed the point. But after about 4 seconds, the pain decreased, and after 10 seconds, when Alice said she felt no discomfort, both the pain of the treatment and that of her lower back had vanished.

Certain types of leg pain are also referred from the gluteals and relieved by pressure there rather than on the legs alone. Usually, the pain that responds to gluteal pressure does *not* include ordinary cramps. As I mentioned in an earlier chapter, cramps require the immediate stretching of the muscle involved. Usually, a dull or throbbing pain in the back of the thigh which seems to originate in the hip will respond dramatically to gluteal finger pressure.

In fact, don't rule out the gluteals when pain is in the lower leg, the upper back, or even the neck. Begin by treating the pressure points closest to the painful area. If relief isn't complete, enlarge the radius of treatment. If your friend feels pain in her neck, treat the neck and head first, then the shoulders, upper and lower back, then the gluteals. When pain is in the lower back or legs, treat the painful area and then move directly to the gluteals.

In general, the primary sites of muscle spasms are the back of the shoulders and the gluteals—you'll find one of those sites involved in an least 75 percent of the cases you treat, no matter where the pain is felt.

In treating gluteal pressure points, you can, and *should* use a great deal of pressure—at least 30 pounds, and some experts advocate even 40 pounds. These muscles, remember, are so strong and relatively insensitive that when they become irritated they usually don't even warn you through localized pain—it's only by the irritation they cause other parts of the body that you suffer at all. To force these pressure points into relaxing will require bullying on your part.

Bullying, but not bruising. Use knuckles, elbow, or even a smoothly rounded stick to get the message across to these gluteal pressure points, but:

- Increase the pressure slowly until you reach maximum force, then maintain that pressure for 10 seconds or until the pain eases.
- Relieve the pressure slowly.
- Do not slide your finger, elbow, or whatever object you're using to create the pressure as you would in classical massage. Simply press downward steadily.
- If relief isn't forthcoming after three or four treatments, have your friend see a doctor.

Pressure Areas of the Buttocks

Area 1. If your job requires a lot of sitting, you can benefit from pressure on the three points of area 1, even if you *don't* have pain. This muscle, known as the gluteus medius, seems to be always under stress, particularly in people who don't exercise. When giving finger pressure massage to treat muscles that are not causing pain, use only *moderate* pressure.

To locate area 1, start with your fingers at the top of the hipbone and slide down about 2 inches. You'll feel a long, cylinder-shaped muscle bulging from the side to about midway across the back, as illustrated. If you have any difficulty locating it, ask your friend to tighten the gluteal muscles, then relax them again before you apply pressure.

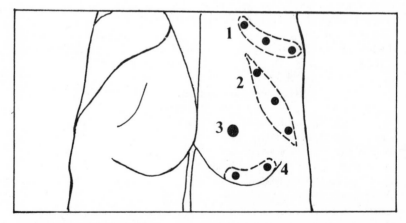

Pressure points in the buttocks are of key importance in relieving pain and tension in the lower back and legs. Area 2, in the hollow of the gluteus maximus, should be given particular attention.

There are *three* pressure points in area 1, and you can treat them individually as you have the others—or, the points are close enough together that, once you're certain you've found the proper locations, you can rest your knuckles across the entire area and apply pressure on all points simultaneously. The key is to make sure that you have located the three pressure points accurately. (There's no benefit in crushing your friend's skin and nerves against her hipbone.)

Area 2. The most crucial pressure points in the gluteals are also the easiest to find. You can usually see the dimpled area on people who exercise regularly even when the muscles are relaxed. If you ask your friend to tighten these muscles, you'll have no difficulty at all. Right in the center of that hollow area is the major pressure point. The other two points are at each extremity of the dimple, as illustrated.

You'll find them easily, for they're always sensitive, which means they're always causing tension—if not pain—elsewhere in the body. In fact, it was this crucial pressure point area that caused Alice's intolerable lower back pain.

Because they're so sensitive, you should begin with soft pressure and increase gradually to heavy pressure.

Area 3. From the lowest pressure point in area 2, move two or three finger thicknesses toward the spine. When you press there you should feel the sacrum and the sacroiliac—not *beneath* your fingers, but *against the side* of the finger closest to the spine. Unless there is severe irritation, you will have to press firmly to locate this point—and there's only one in the area. Area 3 is more often involved in leg pain than in lower back pain.

Area 4. Pain originating in this area can be referred to many parts of the body, and you'd be wise to treat these points when dealing with any complaints in the neck, shoulder, back, and legs.

If you cup your hands around the *bottom* of the gluteus maximus, you'll have an idea of the contour of area 4. The *first* point is just below the rounded tip of the ilium.

If you follow that bone outward to where it joins the femur, or leg bone, you'll find the *second* point. You'll need to use a good deal of pressure in searching this area.

Arms and Hands

The most common ailments of both the upper and lower extremities that frequently can be helped by finger pressure are arthritis, sprains, strains, and ordinary cramps. Because cramps are far more common in the legs than elsewhere, I'll deal with them in the "Legs and Feet" section.

ARTHRITIS

About 22 million Americans have arthritis, and one in seven is at least partially crippled by it. Although it can occur in any joint in the body, the most common areas are those we use most—hands, wrists, elbows, shoulders, hips, knees, and feet.

Actually, *arthritis* is a broad term (like the common cold), covering virtually any pain or inflammation of the joints and the tissues supporting them. The two most common forms are osteoarthritis and rheumatoid arthritis.

Osteoarthritis was long considered an inevitable part of aging. Over the years, the wear and tear in much-used joints finally breaks down the cushion of cartilage that keeps bones apart. Then, the bones themselves rub against each other like machine parts that haven't been oiled. They wear down, creak and grind sluggishly and painfully against each other.

Researchers have recently discovered that osteoarthritis might result in part from dietary deficiencies of the nutrients needed for maintaining strong bones and cartilage. Although there's also probably a genetic component, and certain manual occupations increase chances of developing arthritis, diets lacking in calcium, fluoride, magnesium, phosphorus, and vitamin D play a major role in allowing bones to become brittle and porous.

Another reason that osteoarthritis develops is a lack of exercise. If you've ever thought that those champion weight lifters who hoist 400 pounds and more differ from you and me only because they have more muscle, you're mistaken. They also have more bone—larger and stronger than ours. Otherwise, the extraordinary stress of the muscle pulling against the bone would cause the bone to fracture. (Indeed, that occasionally happens even among trained weight lifters.)

The body in its wisdom strengthens our bones in direct proportion to the stress our muscles place on them. Sedentary people have smaller, weaker bones than active people do, and therefore are more susceptible to the bone degeneration of osteoarthritis over the years.

You can't *cure* osteoarthritis with finger pressure massage. In fact, although the progress of the disease can sometimes be slowed through improved nutrition and a carefully planned exercise program, the only way to reverse serious damage to the joint is to replace it surgically with an artificial one. Finger pressure, remember, is only effective in relaxing cramped or chronically shortened muscles and in relieving pain of muscular origin.

Yet, finger pressure might go a long way toward relieving the *suffering* of the osteoarthritis victim. Here's how:

When movement causes pain for the osteoarthritis victim, he or she avoids it. The unused muscle begins shortening after only a few days of immobility, and after a year or more, those idle muscles lose most of their elasticity. At that point, a slight thoughtless movement can cause excruciating pain, as the muscles contract against the threatening motion, tear, and perhaps pull the joints out of normal alignment. These muscles need to be relaxed and stretched—a combination of finger pressure and classic massage.

Most of those disabled by arthritis suffer the rheumatoid kind. We're not certain what causes it, although current research suggests it might be an autoimmune disease, like an allergy, in which the body in attempting to defend itself overreacts to such an extreme that the defense mechanisms destroy healthy tissue.

In rheumatoid arthritis, the synovial membrane lining the inside of the joint becomes inflamed and swollen, pressing against the bone and forcing the joint to enlarge. That damages and eventually destroys the cartilage, weakens the bone, and strains the ligaments. Even surrounding muscles become inflamed.

Again, finger pressure can't cure rheumatoid arthritis, and neither can any other approach, including drugs, at the moment. Even proper nutrition and exercise can't do much for the rheumatoid sufferer. Steroid drugs, which have dangerous side effects, can bring dramatic relief in some cases, and of course a surgeon can replace the bad joint with a good artificial one.

What finger pressure *can* do is relieve the pain and spasm of the affected muscles, and there are many—both locally and at some distance from the diseased joint—in rheumatoid. In no case should pressure be put on the joint itself, and if your friend reports pain other than that related to normal pressure point sensitivity, *don't treat that area.*

Use good common sense in applying pressure in areas adjacent to damaged joints. You can often get surprisingly good results by relaxing muscles at some distance from the painful area. Perhaps it's the referred pain phenomenon working in reverse: The easing of secondary tension helps the primary muscles to relax as well. For example, you'll find that you can bring noticeable relief to an arthritic hand by massaging pressure points in the forearm and upper arm.

STRAINS AND SPRAINS

A muscle is *strained* when it's overstretched, causing the muscle fibers to tear. As a result of the injury, the muscle will often contract, putting even more stress on the damaged fibers. That can lead to increased pain and swelling.

For a day or two, the muscle shouldn't be used, but if the muscle is large you can relieve tension and thereby reduce the pain by applying finger pressure at points somewhat removed from the injury site. Your friend will tell you when he feels pain other than the usual discomfort of pressure point massage. If he reports such pain, you're too close to the injury.

A *sprain* is more serious than a strain, for it's the tearing of ligaments that connect the muscle to bone, and usually involves bleeding in and around a joint.

Because the pain of the sprain is much more severe than that of a strain, the muscles along the entire limb can go into spasm. When a wrist is sprained, begin searching for pressure points in the shoulder and continue along the arm until you approach the sensitive area. Do *not* use finger pressure near the injury.

To reduce the internal bleeding that will lead to swelling and increased pain, elevate the damaged area and apply ice or a coolant spray. Keep the injured limb immobile until the swelling subsides, then make sure it *is* a sprain and not a broken bone.

Pressure Areas of the Upper Arm

There are many muscles in your arms. There's one to lift your index finger up, another to pull it down, another to move it to the left, another to the right, another to bend it at the first joint, another at the second, and so forth. There are similar muscles in the remaining fingers, and muscles to move your entire hand at the wrist, and at the elbow, and at the shoulder. A discussion of all those muscles and their pressure points would give you far more information than you'll ever need to know.

In this section we'll concentrate on the *primary* muscles and pressure points, those most likely to be the source of pain and stiffness. If treating them doesn't bring sufficient relief, conduct a systematic search for sensitive areas, beginning at the shoulder and working toward the fingers.

THE OUTER ARM

If you allow your arm to hang casually at your side, your open hand flat against your thigh, three sides of your arm are visible to

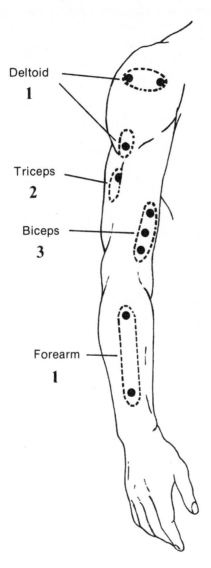

Pressure points along the entire outer arm.

someone standing *beside* you—that's what I refer to as your outer arm. The three major muscle groups in the upper half of the outer arm are the *deltoid, triceps,* and *biceps.*

Area 1. The *deltoid,* or shoulder muscle, (area 1) has three primary pressure points. One is on each side of the humerus, or upper arm bone, just below its connection at the shoulder joint. You'll find both points two or three finger thicknesses below the rise of the humerus. Although the deltoid is a large muscle, these points are sensitive and easy to find.

The third point is not so simple to locate. Hold the outer edge of the deltoid between your thumb and index finger and slide down to its narrowest width—on the outer arm about level with the armpit. The pressure point is here, directly over the humerus.

Area 2. The *triceps* (area 2) is on the back part of the arm, the area where middle-aged sedentary people often discover sagging skin. The easiest way to find the outline of this muscle is to have your friend sit in a chair, place the *back* of his hand against the seat, and press downward. You'll notice that one muscle, the triceps, grows particularly firm.

Have your friend relax the arm. Just below the deltoid, where the triceps seems to slide under the humerus, you'll find the single sensitive pressure point.

Area 3. The *biceps* is the muscle that body builders flex to demonstrate their physiques. The muscle contains three pressure points, and the easiest way to find them is simply by searching. Use a pinching technique, thumb on one side, index finger on the other. Begin at the center—or belly—of the muscle and work toward the elbow to locate the *three points.*

THE INNER ARM

The inner arm is the part facing your friend's body when his arm hangs freely and the palm of his hand rests against his thigh.

Area 1. This area on the inner arm is also one of the most important. It's about an inch beneath the armpit. If you press your thumb into this area and move it from side to side, your friend will probably feel an "electric buzz" along the arm. The sensation won't be a great deal different from bumping his elbow, or funny bone, as it was called years ago. Those are *not* the pressure points —and there are two in this area. Move up into the biceps a finger thickness or two and you'll be on or very close to the points.

Area 2. Area 2, point 1, is behind area 1 along the upper edge of the triceps. Search just behind the bone. The point will be sensi-

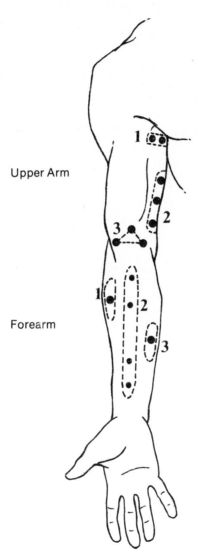

Pressure points along the entire inner arm.

tive. Find the remaining two points by searching along the edge of the muscle toward the armpit.

Area 3. This area includes three points, all of which are sensitive and can be related to pain anywhere along the arm, from shoulder to fingers.

Note that two of the three points in area 3 are slightly below the elbow and are therefore part of the forearm. I'm including them here for convenience.

The first is *just below the elbow* on the thumb side of the arm. If you point your finger at someone, then wag it up and down, you'll feel the muscle harboring this point tighten and relax in the forearm.

Just *above* the elbow and on the inner side of the biceps you'll find the second point.

The final one is on the opposite side of the inner arm from point 1 in this area. It's also just below area 2 of the upper arm.

Pressure Areas of the Forearm

OUTER FOREARM

If you let your arm hang at your side, palm against thigh, the part of your arm visible to someone standing next to you is the outer forearm. There's one pressure point area here, with two points, in addition to the minor ones that you might occasionally need to search out.

You'll find point 1 just below the elbow where the forearm is at its widest. When you try to locate it on a friend, have him relax with his arm at his side while standing and spread his fingers wide. You'll feel the tightening of a long, narrow muscle in the center of the outer part of his forearm. The muscle is in a precise vertical line with the middle finger. Where that muscle bulges at the elbow you'll find the point.

Point 2 is at the narrowest part of the arm, just above the wrist. Find the space between the radius and the ulna, the two bones in the forearm. The pressure point will be hiding there.

THE INNER FOREARM

Area 1. The muscle that contracts when you point your finger and wag it (the brachioradialis, if you're curious), has another pressure point area a few inches below the one at the elbow. It's often so sensitive that you can detect it by searching the muscle along an imaginary line from area 3, point 1, above, to the thumb. Apply moderate pressure in a slow, circular motion. Your friend will tell you when you've touched the point.

Area 2. This area harbors *four pressure points*. As illustrated, they're located precisely in the center of the arm. They're not particularly sensitive unless irritated, so use firm pressure and search at half-inch intervals from elbow joint to wrist.

Area 3. This area is in a plane with the side of the small finger. If you have trouble finding it, locate the ulna, the bone on the small finger side of the forearm. The single pressure point is located in the muscle next to that bone on the inner arm.

Pressure Areas of the Hands

You'll find four major pressure points in the hands, two on the palm side, two on the back.

One is in the heel of the hand above the thumb, and the second is on the back of the hand in the flesh between thumb and index finger. I mention them together because that's how they should

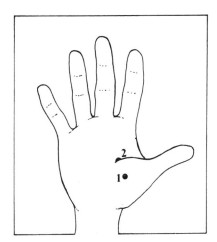
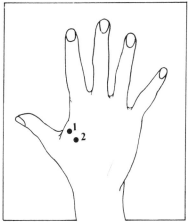

Major pressure points in the hand. Each point on the front of the hand should be pressed simultaneously with the corresponding point on the back.

be searched and pressed, your thumb on one side and your index finger on the other. You'll find that pain in the forearm can often be relieved by pressure at these two points simultaneously.

The second point in the palm is just below the heel. It, too, should be pressed simultaneously with the point on the back of the hand. In fact, it's precisely opposite that point on the back.

The final point on the back of the hand is easy to find. Slide your thumb in the space between the bones of the index finger and the thumb toward the wrist. The point is located in the flesh where the bones intersect.

If you have trouble finding the minor pressure points involved in stiffness and pain, here's a simplified "search and destroy" technique: First, find out which muscle controls the problem area. You can do that by moving the corresponding area on your own body and noting which muscles are involved. For example, raising his forearm with the palm toward his face might create pain in your friend's wrist. But if you move *your* arm the same way, you'll see it's the biceps that actually does the work.

Once you discover which muscles actually control the effort that brings pain, you can assume that the pain is probably referred. Search out the pressure points where the problem actually exists, and apply pressure to the most sensitive areas.

The Legs and Feet

The most active voluntary muscles by far among most people are those in the legs and feet. That should be good news, for we know that muscles can't be healthy unless they're exercised regularly.

And it *is* good news, to a point. The lower extremities are common sites of cramps, strains, sprains, arthritis, stiffness, and reduced range of motion. These conditions strike the hip, knee, ankle, and foot as often as they do the shoulder, elbow, wrist, and hand.

Here are some other frequent causes of pain and injury in the lower extremities, and here's how finger pressure can help.

Pressure Areas of the Thigh

Anytime you hear a complaint of pain in the thigh, you can be reasonably sure that one of two common injuries is at fault. The first is a hamstring pull. The hamstrings—those huge muscles on the back of your thigh—are very hard working. They *contract* (which means they shorten) many times every day. But, unless we're professional football punters or ballerinas, few of us are called upon in the ordinary course of things to *stretch* them. So the muscles grow shorter. Then, we make a sudden move, expecting the muscle to yield. Instead, it either tears or, more commonly, contracts violently in a painful spasm or cramp.

The second most common thigh problem can take months or years to develop. It can be caused by improperly fitting shoes, poor posture, a broken bone in the foot or leg that failed to heal properly —any number of factors that put an abnormal strain on a particular muscle. It might have to work harder than it should to correct a postural imbalance; it might be forced to function in a position that stresses it abnormally.

Finger pressure massage will relieve pain from either condition, but only temporarily. The long-term solution requires more effort. Short muscles should be stretched through regular exercise. You'll find a muscle stretching program in Part IV.

The chronic problems of muscle strain from misuse and overuse might require a more complex solution. If you can't diagnose and solve the problem yourself, you should see an orthopedic physician before the situation becomes irreversible.

Regardless of where your friend *feels* pain in the lower extremities, you should begin by treating the major pressure points in the thigh; often, knee and foot pain is actually caused by spasms in the thigh. Use firm pressure—20 to 30 pounds—for searching and treating these tough muscles.

FRONT OF THE THIGH

Area 1. This area contains only one pressure point. If you stand behind your friend and place the palm of your hand over his hipbone with your fingers parallel to the leg and pointing toward the foot, the tip of your extended thumb should be at the edge of the area. You'll probably have a difficult time finding the pressure point if your friend is standing, however—the pressure point slips beneath connective tissue unless the muscle is completely relaxed. Mark the general area first, then have your friend lie on his back while you search for the point.

Area 2. This area is on the outside of the leg, as indicated in the drawing. Ask your friend to lie on his back and lift his foot, keeping his knee straight. About 6 inches below the hipbone, you'll feel the beginning of an indentation on the outside of the leg that contin-

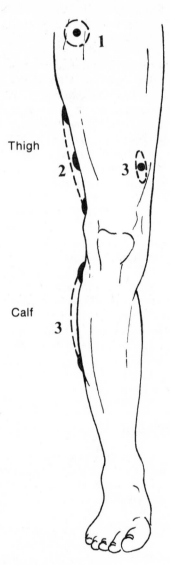

Pressure points along the front of the leg.

ues to the knee joint. Search all along the indentation for pressure points. You'll find one about halfway between the hip and knee, another just above the knee, and a third between the first two.

Area 3. This area has a single pressure point. It's located about 3 inches above the kneecap and to the inside. Fortunately, this is a sensitive point. You can find it easily by sliding your right hand across your friend's right knee and toward his waist, your thumb on one side of the quadriceps (the muscle attached to the knee-cap), and your fingers on the other. As the muscle begins to flare, your thumb will press against the sensitive spot along the side of the quadriceps.

BACK OF THE THIGH

The pressure points I've been detailing are the major ones, the areas of the muscle most likely to spasm when the muscle is "insulted," or traumatized. But the hamstring muscles are always getting insulted, so, in addition to the pressure points I'll discuss, you will often find many more. When the hamstrings are directly involved, treat the major pressure points first, then begin at the gluteals and work your way toward the knee, searching the entire muscle at 1-inch intervals. You'll be surprised at how many more sensitive points you'll find in the hamstrings.

Here are the three areas that harbor the major pressure points:

Area 1. This area is at the gluteals. Try to press in and under the gluteals as you search, beginning at the inside of the thigh.

Area 2. Pressure points in area 2 are located in the center and the extreme edges of the hamstring, but there's considerable variation among people as to the exact location. Search with firm pressure.

Area 3. You'll have an easier time finding the points in area 3. If you put your fingers in the hollow behind your friend's knee, you'll feel two tendinous cords, one on each side of the joint. Follow those cords along the thigh for a distance of approximately two hand-widths. The points are located just on the outside of each cord.

Pressure Areas of the Calf

The gastrocnemius, the major calf muscle, extends along virtually the entire back of the lower leg. You'll find the major

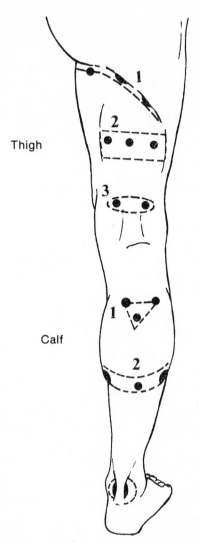

Thigh

Calf

Back of the leg. Area 1 in the thigh can be responsible for referred pain in the back and also the leg. In the calf, pressure area 2 can often relieve lower leg cramps.

pressure points in the muscle's belly, the part that bulges when you stand on your toes. They're along the bottom and top of the belly, and if you press along the outer edges, you'll have no difficulty finding the three points in *area 1* and the three in *area 2*.

You'll also find two points in *area 3*, along the outer edge of the muscle (see drawing).

Pressure Areas of the Foot

For relaxing tired muscles in the calf or foot, find the point behind the Achilles tendon. It's in the soft tissue just above the heel bone (see drawing). If you have difficulty finding this point at first, work deeper into the foot above the heel bone.

There are pressure points between many of the bones of the upper foot, although most of them are minor ones and will prove sensitive only when they have suffered direct injury. Search carefully the soft tissue surrounding the bones and tendons of the upper part of each toe.

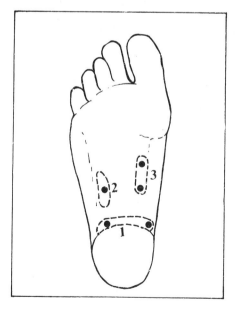

Areas 1, 2, and 3 on the bottom
(sole) of the foot.

Area 1. The bottom part of the foot, or sole, allows much easier access to major foot muscles and pressure points. Area 1 points are located where the heel rises toward the arch. The inner point is at the inner edge of the foot; the outer one is about 1 inch from the outer edge of the foot.

Area 2. This area is in a direct line between the second point in area 1 and the toe next to your little toe. This point is in the very center of the arch.

Area 3. Both points of area 3 are in the arch directly in line with the space between the big toe and the second one. These points are highly sensitive. More than 10 or 12 pounds of pressure here not only will cause pain but can induce a foot cramp as the muscle protectively goes into a spasm.

If your friend has recently begun jogging or exercising and her feet are tired, sore, and aching, you should search out spontaneous pressure points throughout the entire sole, heel, and balls of the toes. Use enough pressure to relax the muscle, but not so much as to cause real pain. How much? A curious thing about the foot is that each point might require a different amount of pressure— a great deal on the heel, for example, much less in certain parts of the arch. You might arrange a wordless signal with your friend. When the pressure reaches the maximum she's willing to endure, have her nod.

When you're treating tired, aching feet with no specific symptoms, it's always wise to include classical foot massage together with finger pressure. That helps to stretch the muscles, keeping the feet from becoming stiff. It also speeds muscle recovery through increased circulation. Chapter 5 includes classical foot massage.

The Chest and Abdomen

The muscles of our bodies are like the interstate highway system near Baltimore: a mass of confusion several layers deep, crisscrossing, intersecting. Some muscles extend left to right, others from top to bottom, and still others from an inner part of the body toward the outer surface.

There's a functional purpose to this, of course (I mean the muscles—I'm not so sure about the highways): We have the ability to move most parts of our bodies in almost any direction we choose. That's particularly true of the torso—the chest and abdomen.

Pressure Areas of the Chest

In the chest we have the large pectorals, the muscles weight lifters work so hard to develop. The latissimus dorsi, the large back muscle we discussed earlier, inserts at the humerus near the armpit to form the fleshy bulge on the side of the chest. This is the muscle that gives the V-shape to some physiques.

Area 1. This area is just below the collarbone. Although there are only two pressure points illustrated, you might find several additional ones in the dotted area. Begin at the shoulder, and search about an inch beneath the clavicle until you reach the first rib.

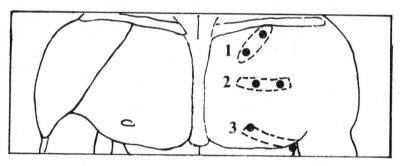

Chest areas 1, 2, and 3.

Area 2. This area is on a plane with the armpits. The first point is about 2 inches from the side of the body, the second 2 more inches toward the sternum.

Area 3. This area has two major pressure points, but, like area 1, there can be several minor ones that need treating. One is at the outside lower edge of the pectorals. The other is at the opposite end of the shaded area, on the same level as the nipple, but about 2 inches closer to the sternum.

About technique: in men, these points can be pressed with 15 pounds of pressure or more using thumbs, knuckles, or even elbows. A good method for the points in area 3 is to grasp the muscle between your thumb and index finger and squeeze firmly. Make sure you have the edge of the pectoral muscle between your fingers, and not merely fat tissue that accumulates here. Squeezing fat and skin will hurt, and it won't do a thing for the muscle.

If your friend is female, don't appiy pressure to the breasts. In most cases, the breast can be moved to one side, the other, and finally upward to give access to all the pressure points; but if the glands are large or firm, you might not be able to reach every area without the risk of bruising breast tissue.

In that case, simply concentrate on treating points in the shoulders, arms, back, and neck. That will help siphon off any referred tension in chest muscles.

Pressure Areas of the Abdomen

The most prominent muscle of the abdomen is the rectus abdominis. There are two of them, one on each side of the centerline of your body (sternum through navel), and they're about as wide as your hand. They originate at the pubic bone, are inserted at the ribs, and cover the center of the abdomen. If you curl your head forward as you do sit-ups, these are the primary muscles that do the work.

The muscle at your sides that wraps around your abdomen is the external oblique. It helps you move your upper body from side to side and at the waist. Beneath that muscle is the internal oblique. Its fibers run at right angles to the muscle above it. A third layer of muscle, the transversus abdominus, is even deeper than the internal oblique and runs horizontally across the abdomen. In the movies, the sergeant who yells, "Suck in your gut, private!" would be technically more accurate to command, "Contract your transversus abdominus!"

Applying finger pressure massage to the abdomen is more difficult than elsewhere for two reasons. First, many vital organs nestle under those abdominal muscles, and too much pressure can bruise them. Second, it's difficult to reach a pressure point in a muscle hidden beneath layers of other muscles without bruising them in the process.

A rule of thumb: Apply only 5 pounds of pressure when you're pushing into the abdomen, and never press when there's pain or discomfort.

Area 1. This area has two pressure points. If you bend your fingers and rest your knuckles in the space between the ilium (hipbone) and ribs, moving them far enough over the abdomen so that the fingers touch but don't rest on the bones, your knuckles will be over this area. One point is near the ribs, the other on a level with the navel.

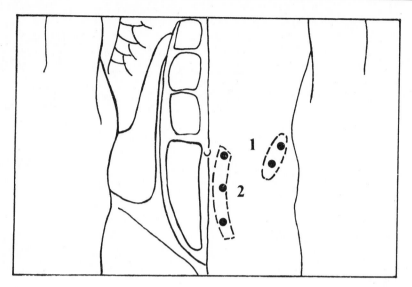

Abdominal areas 1 and 2.

Area 2. This area begins at the navel and extends to about an inch above the pubic bone. Two of the pressure points are at each extreme, and the third is just below midpoint in the shaded area.

Finger pressure massage of the muscles won't cure gas pain, constipation, diarrhea, or other disorders of the digestive tract, but it *will* relieve the tension in the abdominal muscles that inevitably accompanies those conditions. Wait until the condition itself is improved before applying finger pressure massage, and also include classical techniques.

A reminder: Tension in the abdominal muscles is often referred from primary points in the gluteals and lower back. Any pressure point massage of the abdomen should also include those muscle groups.

CHAPTER TEN

ADVANCED FINGER PRESSURE MASSAGE

Thus far, we've concentrated on finger pressure massage for functional ailments, everyday aches and pains that may not be severe enough to require medical attention but which are troublesome nevertheless. In this chapter, you'll learn about various forms of advanced finger pressure massage which are designed to be used in conjunction with a doctor in treating more serious problems. We'll be looking specifically at deep friction massage for preventing scar tissue buildup after an injury or an operation, and visceral healing techniques—shiatsu, connective tissue massage, and reflexology—for the treatment of organic illness.

The important thing to remember here is that these are techniques that you should be using in addition to medical treatment, not in place of it, in dealing with your friend's condition or illness. And because they are advanced types of finger pressure massage, you may find them difficult to do by yourself; in this case, you and your friend may want to seek the aid of a professional physical therapist who is trained in these techniques.

Deep Friction Massage

If you've ever had surgery—or even if you've just cut yourself—you know what a scar feels like. You know that it doesn't stretch unless you force it to, and that's painful. Enough scar tissue in the wrong place can make you an invalid.

That fact is the crux of one of the most exciting and promising massage techniques: deep friction. The practitioner of this technique—usually a physical therapist—uses finger pressure, but doesn't seek out pressure points. Instead, he or she concentrates on scar tissue.

According to James H. Cyriax, the leading proponent of deep friction, manual friction applied in the right way to the right spot "can secure quick and permanent successes unequalled by any other means known today." In that sweeping statement Cyriax includes drugs and the most expensive equipment in the physical therapist's armory. Yet, in specific cases, Cyriax is entirely correct.

Those cases involve tears in muscle fibers. The tear might be in the "belly" of the muscle—usually its thickest part—or where the muscle attaches to the tendon.

The usual pressure point techniques described in previous chapters will relieve the *pain* of muscle ruptures by helping the muscle to relax but they don't prevent scar tissue buildup. The sliding strokes of classical massage, always in the direction of the muscle fibers, aid in circulation, but again don't affect scar tissue. Deep friction alone can help.

When a muscle is torn, new fibrous—or scar—tissue begins to form almost immediately. The scar tissue might be compared with a first-aid glue that the body produces; a tough patch that stops the bleeding, eases the pain, and holds the damaged tissue together. It works fine as long as you don't try to use the muscle, for scar tissue itself is relatively insensitive to pain—and it's not very flexible.

When a healthy muscle contracts, its fibers shorten and spread out, causing the muscle to bulge. Scar tissue is unable to spread, however, so any effort to use the muscle can be very painful. Thus we restrict our range of motion.

Many people who have written themselves off as arthritics because any movement beyond a limited range is painful are actually victims of muscle scarring. They can be helped with deep friction massage.

Let's continue to visualize the scar tissue as a clump of glue, and let's imagine the healthy fibers growing to unite the torn muscle as strands of hair. You wouldn't succeed in removing that glue and freeing the hair by rubbing the glue in the direction the strands grow. To free the strands, you must rub *across* the hair, breaking the strands away from each other.

The unique thing about deep friction massage is that *it's always done in transverse* fashion, or at right angles to the muscle fibers.

In the words of James Cyriax, "adhesions in muscle can be

broken, not by stretching, but only by forceably broadening the muscle out."

It's best to begin deep friction massage as soon as an injury begins healing, because if it's done properly and regularly, excess accumulation of fibrous tissue can be prevented in the first place. But the technique can also break down long-standing fibrous tissue. It will just take more sessions—and cause more discomfort.

Unfortunately, deep friction massage is *always* somewhat painful, just as separating your hair from the glue would be. You can reduce the discomfort significantly by relaxing the muscle before treatment. You wouldn't try to remove glue from your hair by pulling the strands taut and applying firm sideward pressure— you might well pull the hair right out of your head. The same is true of a muscle receiving deep friction.

Another reason the muscle must be relaxed: If it's tight, your finger will slide *over* the muscle, not rub the fibers against each other, which is essential to breaking up the scar tissue.

FINDING THE SPOT

Now that you understand how deep friction works, you can see that knowing precisely where the scar tissue exists is absolutely essential to effective treatment. Says Cyriax, "Before accurate massage can be administered to a lesion, its situation and extent must first have been defined to within a finger's breadth by the doctor's diagnosis." Cyriax apparently believes that it will be almost impossible for anyone untrained in anatomy and physiology to pinpoint the precise area of injury. We've already discussed the difficulty of pinpointing the source of pain—pain in one part of the body can be referred from an injury elsewhere, whereas the injury site itself seems to be free of pain. We can't assume that where it hurts is where we should apply pressure.

Another reason Cyriax would like deep friction massage left to the professional physical therapist working in conjunction with a physician is that untrained people don't know *which* layer of muscle is injured. In some parts of the body (the abdomen is a good example) muscle stretches across muscle several layers thick, the fibers of no two of them running in the same direction. If an amateur misdiagnosed a scar in the external oblique and treated it with deep friction to the rectus abdominus, his pressure would be too superficial to do anything significant for the muscle that was injured—and the strokes would be in the wrong direction.

These are valid points, of course. That doesn't necessarily mean that you shouldn't attempt deep massage when it's appropriate. It *does* mean, especially when the injury is serious (a bad strain or an involvement of tendons or ligaments), that you should:

- Work closely with a physician to identify the *exact* location of the injury, including the depth of the muscle involved and the direction of its fibers. (Remember, fibers usually run in the same direction as the part of the body they move when contracting.)
- Follow directions exactly.
- Seek a professional physical therapist to apply deep friction massage when the injury is serious or particularly painful to the touch—or if you achieve no positive response within a few days.

In general, you can identify the muscle involved by noting what sort of movement causes pain. For example, let's assume you have a severe pain in the biceps of the upper arm, with sensitive pressure points from wrist to shoulder. Is the problem really in the biceps? To test that, bend your arm at the elbow and clench your fist. The biceps will contract—and the pain will probably increase.

But other muscles in your arm also contracted. Now, straighten your arm and clench your fist again. This time, only one muscle contracts—the flexor digitorum of the forearm. And with that movement, the pain grows sharper. So, you've tracked down the muscle where the injury actually exists, sparing yourself useless and painful effort.

It'll take patience and a good understanding of the body's musculature to learn which muscles are actually involved. First, determine the *direction of movement* that causes the pain—or the greatest pain—because any number of movements can be painful in some muscle ruptures. Then, find out *which specific muscle* contracts to cause that precise movement. Remember that muscles do work by contracting only, pulling their two extremes closer together. The fibers that compose pectoral muscles of the chest, for example, extend from the clavicle and sternum to the shoulder area. You can see that these fibers contract to pull the upper arm inward, lift it upward, and even press it downward. But for all their strength, they're completely useless for outward pressure. If that movement causes the pain, you're wasting time on the pectorals if you give them deep friction.

When you're certain you've found the right muscle, search it as you would for pressure points. And let's give your friend some credit for having a brain. You might ask him or her where it hurts, and he or she might just tell you. It's highly unlikely that the spot your friend identifies is precisely correct. It's like having an itch, yet not quite being able to scratch the right spot. When your friend directs you to the approximate area, begin searching, relatively gently, for the primary pain area.

LIGAMENTS

Most ligaments connect bone to bone. We usually find them at joints, and when they're damaged serious problems can result—including crippling. Proper treatment should be given by trained professionals. Their job is to prevent adhesions from developing in the joint area—which would be like throwing glue on a door hinge. At the same time, they must avoid stretching the ligament so that it fails to keep the bone properly aligned. Unless you have such training, I recommend that you do not use deep friction on ligament injuries.

You can, however, provide a real service by using frequent classical sliding and *superficial* friction on the injured area. That will help to reduce swelling and disperse blood clots, significantly speeding recovery.

MUSCLE STRAINS

A muscle strain is a tear. Allow a day or two for the healing to get underway as new tissue begins uniting the torn muscle fibers. When you do begin massaging, use light pressure to avoid breaking those new connections. The goal is simply to keep these new tissue strands from sticking to each other and forming a solid scar lump.

Use one finger—your index or middle finger—on small areas. Larger areas and deeper muscles might require use of three inner fingers bunched together.

Make sure before you begin the stroke that the muscle is *passively* contracted—that is, your friend's limb is contracted to the extreme that the muscle *would* bring it, but without the muscle doing the work. In that position, although the muscle is completely relaxed, it is short and spread out, the fibers naturally separating from each other—yet loose so that your finger can manipulate the new tissue.

Begin your stroke at one side of the muscle and move across the strained area to the opposite side. Your fingers should *not* slide over the skin; rather, the deeper tissues of the skin should slide against the muscle fibers.

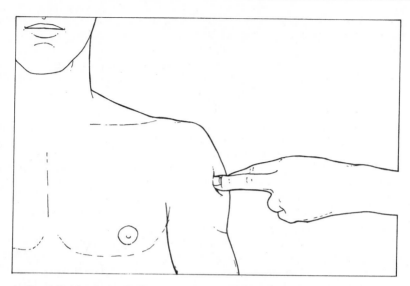

In the deltoid muscle, fibers run from the shoulder bone in the direction of the elbow. In deep friction massage, the muscle should be thoroughly relaxed and the strokes should move in short, deep strokes at a right angle to the muscle fibers to loosen the scar tissue that holds those fibers together.

Unlike the pressure point techniques described in previous chapters, the deep massage stroke is not so much downward as it is *sideward*. It's not the pressure alone that separates new fibers from each other but the *rolling* of them against each other.

The speed of the stroke should be brisk and sweeping.

If the strain has long since healed and the resulting scar tissue makes full range of movement painful, you must use a somewhat different technique to break up the adhesion. You'll need to apply a good deal more pressure, because you're actually ripping the deep-seated scar tissue apart. It will certainly be painful for your friend. You can ease that pain to a great degree by searching out the pressure points in the surrounding muscle tissue and treating them with the usual finger pressure. Within three to five minutes —all that's necessary for a single treatment—your friend should notice some improvement in range of movement.

Finally, let me emphasize again that you can do your friend harm by using this forceful technique on a misdiagnosed ailment (a tumor, for example), or in areas that are inaccurately pin-pointed. For those reasons, it's essential to have a physician see your friend first if the complaint is potentially serious.

VISCERAL HEALING MASSAGE

There are several types of massage whose practitioners claim to treat disorders of the inner organs—the heart, lungs, liver, and such. The potential of this visceral healing, according to many of its practitioners, is virtually limitless. They believe it effective against heart attacks, headaches, hemorrhoids, cancer, impotence, constipation—virtually every ailment known to humans.

To most Western medical doctors, and laypersons as well, such claims seem impossible. Most headaches are caused by tension, impotence by psychogenic factors, heart attacks by smoking, or poor eating habits or the degeneration of sedentary life-styles. Cancer is a deviation in normal cell proliferation triggered by such factors as toxic chemicals or viruses. How could a single therapy, and a simple one at that, involving nothing more than finger pressure—no costly drugs or hospital gadgets—be effective against all ailments when their causes are so varied?

The answer given by visceral healers is that Western medicine operates with limited vision. Visceral healing methods usually have as their starting point a philosophy of man and nature that differs from traditional Western views. That includes theories on human physiology and the natural sciences for which there is no proof and often precious little evidence.

Yet, as the truism has it, you can't argue with success. Anyone who reads a newspaper knows that even Western medical researchers have recently documented remarkable successes with acupuncture—and shiatsu is the massage version of acupuncture, with its own very long history of remarkable results. In fact, every visceral healing technique has its adherents who claim dramatic healings.

Three of the most popular visceral healing methods are shiatsu, connective tissue massage and, reflexology, and I'll survey each in the following sections. I urge you to approach these pages with a thoughtful, open mind, weighing the techniques and the rationale with those you've already learned and perhaps used. There's much you can gain from them, whether or not you accept the theories that have been constructed to explain their effectiveness.

On the other hand, it would be a possibly disastrous mistake to use visceral healing *in place of* accepted medical techniques when your friend is suffering from a potentially serious ailment. Perhaps you remember the California child who suffered a malignant tumor that in the early stages could have been removed with no serious consequences. She died because she was treated exclusively with visceral healing techniques. Although that was one of the most widely publicized cases, there are many like it every year.

The best approach is to work *with* a doctor in helping to treat your friend's condition or illness.

Shiatsu

Shiatsu, the ancient Japanese adaptation of Chinese techniques, is the original finger pressure massage. Literally, the Japanese *shi* means finger and *atsu* is pressure.

The basic premise of shiatsu is much broader than its health applications. In fact, it's a philosophy of life, a way of viewing people and the universe, and it is a perspective on humankind that is poetic, spiritual, broad, and humble. The Oriental considers each person as part of nature—not in some vague spiritual sense, but literally, *physically*. According to the Oriental view, *ch'i,* the life energy, flows freely through all living things, whether plant, animal, or human, and in this respect the universe is one. But the universe is thought to be united in another aspect as well: Our bodies are composed of precisely the same substances that make up the world around us. These substances are plant (symbolized as wood), heat (fire), earth (the earth), mineral (metal), and liquid (water). In the West, we hold that the world is composed of animal, mineral, and vegetable; in the Orient, they prefer these five divisions, which in turn correspond to parts of the body. Specifically, the heart is related to fire; the kidneys to water; the liver to plant; the spleen to earth; and the lungs to metal.

Those are the major, dominant organs, but each has a passive organ without which it cannot function adequately. For the liver, the passive organ is the gallbladder; for the heart, it's the small intestine. The stomach works with the spleen, the urinary bladder with the kidneys, the large intestine with the lungs.

Traditionally there was another set of organs. The heart constrictor was a protective sac surrounding the heart, which should be understood today in a figurative sense. Its passive counterpart, called the triple-heat, can be thought of as the warming effect of the blood circulation, always present as long as there is life.

These organs cannot function unless they are infused with a constant circulation of *ch'i,* the life force, which flows through the body along a *meridian* system, a network of 14 meridian lines that together reach to all parts of the body.

THE YANG LINES

There are six yang, or positive meridian, lines. They're named after these organs: large intestine, small intestine, stomach, bladder, triple heat, and gallbladder. The energy flow through the yang meridians—and through these organs—begins at the top of your head or your fingertips and flows *downward, toward* your feet— although some lines end in the center of the body.

THE YIN LINES

The associated organs are the major ones—the lung, spleen, kidney, heart, heart constrictor, and liver. *Ch'i* flows through these meridians *from* the toes and center of the body *toward* the head and fingertips.

That accounts for 12 meridian lines. The final two are the major conduits through which the energy flows to all the other meridians. These are called the Governing Vessel Meridian (yang) and the Conception Vessel Meridian (yin).

At various points along all the meridian lines are *tsubos*. The tsubos might loosely be compared with the strainers in a sink. Any body injury or abuse, insults from the environment, and ordinary disease processes "clog up" one or more tsubos like food particles in the strainer, and the flow of *ch'i* is reduced in that area. A sick organ can affect tsubos along that organ's meridian line—and tsubos clogged for reasons unrelated to the organ can nonetheless cause the organ to become ill.

And because all the organs are interrelated through the meridian system, illness anywhere has to have some effect on the entire body.

About 1000 tsubos have been identified, with about 365 commonly recognized. Only 60 to 90 tsubos are used by most practitioners. Each tsubo is about the size of a fingertip.

A shiatsu diagnosis can be made in one of two ways: Your friend might have a complaint, a headache, for example. Those with a knowledge of shiatsu (or those who own or buy a shiatsu text— even the simplest ones are 80 to 150 pages long) will find that they can relieve headaches by applying finger pressure to tsubo 11 and 15, or stomach 36, or gallbladder 20, or bladder 10, 13, and 60, or large intestine 4 and 11, or liver 3—or all of the above.

As you can see, shiatsu is not a simple technique that you can learn overnight. In fact, in the Orient, it's a full-fledged medical speciality that requires years of training. In addition to learning the meridian lines, the expert must be able to find all the tsubos involved—and there are some special tsubos *not* located on meridians.

The second diagnostic approach is used when your friend has

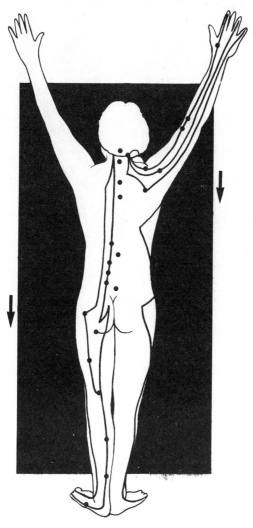

The yang meridians and the tsubos along them. Ch'i flows from the fingertips and head toward the feet.

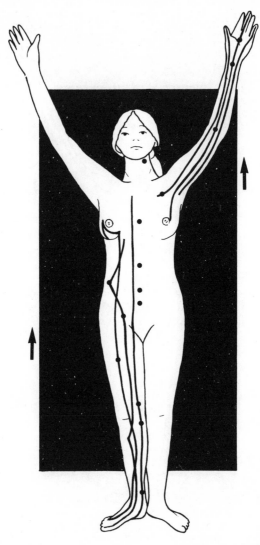

The yin meridians and the tsubos along them. Ch'i flows from the toes toward the head and fingertips.

no symptoms. Tsubos throughout the body are pressed, and any that are highly sensitive indicate blockage. When a painful tsubo is discovered, all the tsubos along that meridian line should be searched, because usually more than one is involved.

As with the other advanced finger pressure techniques, make sure to work in conjunction with a doctor if you are using shiatsu to help treat an organic illness.

As Wataru Ohashi urges in his book, *Do-It-Yourself Shiatsu,* ". . . as a beginner you should never try to cure disease with shiatsu alone. Always consult a doctor if you suspect a friend is seriously ill . . ."

HOW TO PRESS THE TSUBO
Your friend should lie on the floor completely relaxed with no pillow under his head. Place the ball of your thumb directly on the tsubo. Keep your arms straight and use the weight of your body to apply the pressure—and only when your friend is exhaling.

Most tsubos should be pressed for 7 seconds, but those in the tough back muscles require 10 seconds. Although the pressure will cause pain, it should never be even close to intolerable—sharp pain suggests a condition that needs medical attention.

The desired reaction is captured in the Pennsylvania Dutch expression, "It hurts good."

The pressure should be applied gradually and released gradually. Sudden pressing and releasing can cause muscle spasm.

The drawings on pages 153 and 154 illustrate the approximate locations of the tsubos along the meridians. In general, begin your search for sensitive tsubos at the extremities and work toward the center of the body.

Connective Tissue Massage

Elizabethe Dicke, who in 1929 developed a major new method of massage called *Bindegewebsmassage* (connective tissue massage), might never have made the breakthrough had she herself not suffered a serious illness. It started with an infected tooth. The bacteria spread throughout her body and attacked the arteries of her right leg, causing an endarteritis obliterans—an infection that led to a circulatory blockage. As the disease progressed, her leg became cold and grayish-white. The toes began to look gangrenous. The doctor recommended leg amputation.

Dicke was bedridden for five months, during which she also developed severe back pain. As a physical therapist trained in zone therapy, she treated the back pain herself. She wrote in her book, *My Connective Tissue Massage:*

> While lying on my side I palpatated a densely filtrated tissue over the sacrum and iliac crest and on the left side opposite this an increased tension of the skin and the subcutaneous tissue.
>
> I tried to disperse the tension by pulling the strokes in those regions which were hyperesthetic (extremely sensitive to pain). The tension subsided slowly; the back pains disappeared under the relaxing strokes and a strong feeling of warmness set in. After several trials I felt a constant alleviation of my complaint.
>
> Now pins and needles started in my involved leg as far down as the sole, with alternating waves of warmth. The extremity improved constantly. Then I added strokes of the regions over the right greater trochanter (the upper part of the thighbone) and the lateral aspect of the thigh.
>
> Over a three-month period of treatment the severe manifestations of my disease regressed completely. The treatment continued over a longer period of time by one of my colleagues; after one year I could resume fully my activities as physical therapist.

Dicke felt that by massaging her back she had initiated the healing of her leg, and also countered other symptoms she had suffered in vital organs. Thirty years earlier, an English neurologist named Head had described areas on the body which affect specific organs—similar to the shiatsu tsubos. Dicke's connective tissue massage relies on these *Head's Zones* to produce a reflex influence on the vital organs.

Although that idea wasn't new, Dicke did make two original and valuable contributions to massage. The first was her stroke, deep friction using primarily the middle finger—the same technique later used in deep friction massage (see pp. 144–149). And Dicke concentrated on massaging the *connective tissues* that encapsulate the muscles, organs, blood vessels, and other tissues, hold them in place, and attach them to the skeleton. Connective tissue actually holds the entire body together like a fine netting, and Dicke believed that the reflex paths are located in this material.

When the connective tissue thickens, loses its elasticity, or adheres to the surrounding tissues over which it should normally glide smoothly, the result is stiffness, pain, and abnormal reflex effects elsewhere in the body. The solution is to break up the adhesions and restore the connective tissue to a normal state. According to CTM practitioners, that can be done through a massage technique that mechanically tears the connective tissue from that to which it has adhered. At the same time, the stroke, which is an irritation to the tissue, dramatically increases the circulation to the area. "This circulatory response is eventually responsible for adaptive alterations in the 'consistency of the tissue," according to Maria Ebner, British professor of education. Through this improved circulation, the connective tissue regains its normal shape and elasticity.

WHEN TO USE CTM

In Germany, where CTM is very popular, it is used not in place of but in conjunction with traditional medical practices. Most doctors frequently recommend CTM when they feel it will be helpful for vague aches and pains and stiffness. Although CTM practitioners might contribute to therapy for serious ailments, they do so in cooperation with and at the request of the physician in charge.

In America, too, doctors—particularly young ones—are much more willing to take a holistic approach to healing. That means that they will incorporate into treatment healthful approaches that consider the body as a whole. If your friend would like you to treat him for a serious illness using CTM, find a doctor who holds this view and treat your friend strictly within the guidelines he or she establishes.

APPLYING CTM

Unlike other massage methods, both you and the one receiving CTM should be seated.

The finger to use is the middle one, with your ring finger placed on top of the middle fingernail to increase the strength and firmness of the pressure. How much pressure you use depends on the depth of the tissue you're trying to reach. Your finger should *never* slide over the skin, but, as in all friction, should force the underlying tissue to slide across the connective tissue.

You can alter the depth of your stroke by changing the angle of your finger. The closer to a right angle with the tissue your finger is, the deeper the pressure will be.

If you try to use the strength in your fingers, hand, or wrist, you'll achieve about three strokes before your muscles become exhausted and you'll have to quit. Keep your finger, hand, and wrist straight and let the muscles in your arms and body do the work.

You'll know the massage is working when your friend reports a cutting, tearing, or scratching sensation as the connective tissue spearates from that surrounding it. Although this can be painful, it should not be intolerable. Each stroke is a matter of pressing downward, moving your finger to pull the underlying tissue taut, then forcing it a little farther to tear it loose. The entire stroke may cover no more than an inch or two.

FREQUENCY AND DURATION

Because each stroke covers so little distance, an entire CTM for a single localized area might take as much as 45 minutes. Every part of the area must be massaged, preferably with shingling, or overlapping strokes. In the early stages, you should give the massage at least three times a week—daily if you prefer. Later, once or twice a week will be sufficient.

If there's no improvement within two weeks, CTM probably won't help that particular condition. It's time for your friend to ask the doctor for alternative diagnoses and treatments.

Reflexology

In 1913, Dr. William H. Fitzgerald (an American) claimed that by massaging the feet he could bring relief to all parts of the body. Fitzgerald's technique was similar in theory to Chinese finger pressure/acupuncture, but Fitzgerald named his approach *zone therapy*. Today, massage of the feet in efforts to produce changes elsewhere in the body is called reflexology.

Reflexology assumes that there are zones or reflex points in the feet that relate to and dramatically affect the entire body. Therefore, ailments can be diagnosed by locating sensitive spots in the foot. The masseur uses primarily his thumbs and knuckles to apply pressure, section by section, over the entire foot, and when he discovers a tender area, he applies deep—and painful—pressure in that particular location.

Through charts and training, the masseur knows which part of the foot needs attention if a patient has a specific complaint, from poor eyesight to kidney failure. A typical reflexology treatment will take approximately 10 minutes per foot.

The accompanying drawing (page 160) will make it simple for you to try reflexology if you wish. If your friend complains of lower back pain, for example, you'll find the related area on the outside of the upper foot, forward of the heel. Apply firm pressure on that precise spot for 8 to 10 seconds, as you would in ordinary finger pressure massage.

A point often overlooked by authors on the subject is that, if a friend is sitting with her foot on a stool, the sole facing you, you must make sure that her knee joint, too, is supported. The knee should be slightly bent, with a pillow placed beneath it. Otherwise, pressure on her foot can cause the knee to straighten and the ligaments and muscles surrounding it to be severely strained.

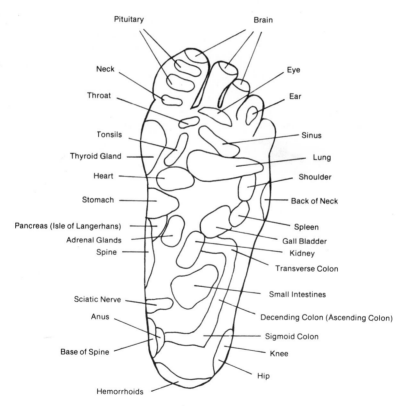

Reflex coordinates of the left foot. Although most reflex points are found in both feet, there are some exceptions. Those parts of the anatomy in parentheses (Island of Langerhans and ascending colon) are located as indicated, but only on the right foot.

PART IV
AIDS TO MASSAGE

CHAPTER ELEVEN

WHAT TO EXPECT FROM MASSAGE AIDS

One writer on massage has suggested that the perfect society would include a robot masseur capable of performing all types of massage 24 hours a day. Frankly, it strikes me as a dreadful idea. If the only value of massage was in getting our tissues jostled and jiggled, the subways would have made masseurs extinct long ago.

Massage is the laying on of *hands*. I have placed my hands on the shoulders of people who have been so tense for so long that their muscles had simply forgotten how to relax. And, over a period of 15 or 20 minutes, with no movement on my part, just the firm touch of hand to body, the tension flowed out of those muscles. Relaxation came, followed by sleep.

I've watched other talented hands relieve long-suffered pain, make depressed people content, and lonely people happy. As I mentioned in the opening chapter, I've seen the miracle of massage. Fifty percent, more or less, was a mechanical effect. The rest was the result of communication between compassionate hands and bodies in need of them.

No mechanical device should ever take the place of hand-to-flesh communication. However, the aids *do* have a place. And when they're used to augment massage rather than to replace it, they can be very satisfying—and sometimes beneficial to health.

I ought to explain what I mean by an aid to massage so that you'll understand why I don't recommend some so-called aids later. An aid is a device, facility, or technique that enhances or prolongs the benefits of a massage.

Now, jogging is a wonderful activity. Some people will live

longer if they jog, and all joggers will feel better as their bodies operate at peak efficiency. But jogging doesn't increase or prolong the benefits of massage.

Stretch exercises, on the other hand, keep the muscles loose and supple. If massage is a first-aid approach to muscle stiffness, stretch exercises are the long-term therapy. That's why I devote Chapter Fourteen to a program of stretch exercises that will keep your muscles loose and your steps springy.

It's the same story with equipment and mechanical devices. I don't know anyone who believes that barbells, for example, will improve the effects of massage; but that doesn't mean you ought not to lift weights. Similarly, you can find a number of devices on the market that are believed to be useful as massage aids but simply aren't, yet they might have other advantages such as providing pleasant sensations and giving a psychological lift. In the following chapter we'll discuss these together with equipment and devices that are of real benefit to massage.

And keep in mind that it isn't necessary to go out and spend money to reap the advantages of some massage aids. You can rely on your own inventiveness to duplicate the effects of some of these devices. For example, a gently applied rolling pin can produce virtually the same effect as some of the equipment we'll discuss in the next chapter. A hot water bottle can substitute for an electric heat pad. And, with one or two exceptions, your hands can learn to do it all.

CHAPTER TWELVE

MECHANICAL EQUIPMENT

Many of you will be surprised, and a few disappointed, about what you're going to learn in this chapter. We'll be discussing many kinds of equipment—vibrators, vibrating belts and beds, whirlpools, and roller devices. Some will be useful to you in giving massage; most, unfortunately, are of little or no use, at least for that purpose. It doesn't mean that you can't go on enjoying them, only that they won't aid in massage.

On the other hand, we'll discuss some devices that can provide benefits which you can't duplicate with your hands. (Try competing with a whirlpool, for example.) They are not essential; you can give a perfectly satisfactory massage without them. Just think of them as the frosting on the cake, and if you have access to them, give them a try.

The Vibrators

The first massage aid that comes to most minds is the vibrator. There are many types of vibrators so, it's important that you know which ones to use—and not to use—under various circumstances.

THE PHALLIC VIBRATORS
In this day and age, there's no need to go into detail about these dime-store novelties. (They're actually priced from about $5 to

$40.) They're usually constructed of an inflexible plastic, although some are made of a pliant latex. Virtually the entire unit vibrates. However, the shape of these units makes them practically useless for real body massage regardless of claims in advertising.

Except for the cheapest models, which keep breaking, they can be fun in sensual/erotic massage. That's what they're actually designed for. Keep these cautions in mind, however: (1) overzealous use can cause chafing on sensitive membranes, and the chafed area can later become infected; (2) too much pressure on the glans or clitoris can cause pain instead of pleasure; (3) prolonged vibration can have an anesthetic effect, making fulfillment difficult or impossible.

PISTOL-GRIP VIBRATORS

These devices usually have interchangeable heads, only two of which are useful to me, personally. The first is the brush head, with scores of tiny rubber nipples or bristles. There's no better way to give a scalp massage if the mechanical effect is all you want. I doubt even the most expert masseur could leave a scalp tingling like these plastic fingers can.

I also use the knob head as an adjunct to finger pressure massage, as a prelude to the finger pressure itself, when the muscle is so tight that I know a great deal of pressure will be needed to effect relief. About two minutes of vibration with the knob head directly on the pressure point anesthetizes it, and sometimes it helps the muscle to relax. The point still needs to be treated, but less forcefully, and my friend feels less discomfort.

The knob head is very useful on the feet, as in reflexology. Here, the muscles are always tight, and you can use very firm pressure with the vibrator as a prelude to massage.

Unfortunately, in spite of these benefits, the pistol-grip vibrator is probably the single most important reason that people who experiment with massage don't find it as gratifying as it can be. Perhaps because it's easy and we're lazy, perhaps because we're a gadget-oriented society, or perhaps just because we don't *know* how to use our hands on our friend's body, many people pass off a full-body vibration as a massage. As you know by now, even manual vibration is appropriate only occasionally, and by itself could never produce the overall benefits and pleasures of a good massage. When the pistol vibrator is used, it must be for a specific purpose only—and then put aside.

THE HAND VIBRATOR

The type of vibrator I find best overall is the one that's held to the back of my hand by straps or springs. It causes my *hands* to vibrate as they massage my friend's body. With one of these on each hand, I can give a typical full-body classical massage while my friend enjoys the added dimension of the vibration.

Using this type of vibrator will take getting used to. You'll have to *concentrate* on the strokes rather than being distracted by your vibrating hands. And, as your hands grow numb from the vibration (and they will) you'll have to keep your mind on what your hands are doing. At first, a 10- to 15-minute massage using these vibrators is about all you should ask of yourself. They're a great help in mini-massages of the neck, shoulder, and back when muscle tension is the main complaint.

THE VIBRATING BED

Unless you were wealthy, for many years you could experience a vibrating bed only by spending a night in a motel or hotel that offered them. Then, if you had enough quarters, you could vibrate all night long. In recent years, however, companies have begun marketing vibration attachments at reasonable cost, and now you can find them in bedrooms all over the country. They *do* help people to relax and sleep better. By easing away tension, they're a nice prelude to massage. But, once again, vibration is not massage, and these beds provide nothing remotely like a real massage.

VIBRATING BELTS

Vibrating (or oscillating) belts, usually found in health clubs and spas, would be equally appropriate in an amusement park. They rarely provide even muscle relaxation, because the vibration is so frantic that the muscles tend to contract protectively. They're used primarily to jiggle fat loose, which is physiological nonsense. Even if the fat *could* be broken down, it could leave the body only as spent energy through exercise. Otherwise, it would be redeposited in precisely the same areas, the fat storage centers—the hips, abdomen, buttocks, and thighs primarily.

The vibrating belt can be beneficial in that it provides a mild form of entertainment akin to a carnival's Tilt-A-Whirl ride—pleasant feelings and perhaps psychological relaxation.

The Whirlpool

There are two types of whirlpools, the bathtub variety and the large, whole-body type.

The bathtub whirlpool is a step above a toy. If it generated the speed of water movement necessary to actually "massage" your body, the water would soar out of your tub and flood your house. The most that can be said for them is that they provide a pleasant and amusing sensation.

The whole-body whirlpool, on the other hand, has proven itself where it really counts, in the locker rooms and gymnasiums used by professional athletes. The heat can relax strained muscles as well as cramped and weary ones, and increase the circulation to speed recuperation. Simultaneously, the forcefully circulating water really does massage the body, although not nearly as effectively as human hands would.

Overall, the whirlpool, if the unit is capable of moving the water with extreme speed, is the next best thing to a genuine massage. I always try to check into a hotel that has one when I'm on the road and my massage partner is far away.

Miscellaneous Devices

There are many gadgets on the market—and some gimmicks—that more or less effectively encourage relaxation and ease muscle tension. If they provide massage, as some of the manufacturers claim, it's only in the loosest meaning of that word.

SHOWER MASSAGERS

Some of these shoot high-pressure pulsating streams of water at the user to produce an effect similar to the striking stroke of manual massage. Another common shower head vibrator incorporates bristles that pulsate at a thousand times a minute to actually massage in combination with the hot water.

These units are particularly useful when pain or stiffness is localized. Whole-body benefits are dubious, however, because it's not possible to relax and lose yourself in the massage. Some muscles must always be at work directing the shower head—or moving the body—to bring the stream of water to another muscle area. Even soaking in the tub doesn't solve the problem.

FOOT RELAXERS

In recent years, several companies have been offering devices to relax the feet. One of the most sophisticated is a small foot tub that the user fills with hot water. In some models, the temperature is maintained by electric coils in the unit. The user inserts his feet, throws a switch, and the floor of the tub vibrates.

After a long day of shopping, few experiences can be as joyful as sitting in front of the television with your feet soaking in warm water that *stays* warm. Some people might enjoy the vibration as well, although it will probably have more effect on the muscles of the calves than of the feet as the vibration radiates up the tibia. These foot tubs are a good remedy for tired feet, but a faster and more thorough one is to have a friend who knows how to give foot massage go to work on you.

Foot rollers actually *do* massage the stubborn muscles on the bottom of your feet. The device is nothing more than a few rows of rolling knobs close enough together to press into every part of your foot. As your foot moves over them (you decide how much pressure to apply), the knobs press everywhere. Obviously, a friend's fingers can seek out points that need special attention. They can also spread your foot, tug the toes, and accomplish so many subtle pleasures that no gadget can duplicate. As a standby, though, the foot roller is as good as any other device to relieve tired feet.

CHAPTER THIRTEEN

SAUNA AND STEAM

If you were to read of several men cramped into a tiny room with bare wooden walls and floor, no furniture except wooden bunks and heated to 200°F by glowing rocks, you'd probably think it a form of torture. In fact, that scene is enacted by hundreds of thousands of Americans every day—a typical sauna bath.

In Finland, the sauna is as old as the country's recorded history. Sauna originated there, and even today, a typical Finnish home-builder constructs a sauna even before completing the house to which it will be attached. There are nearly a million saunas in Finland today—not counting those built in the woods or near the country's 100,000 lakes and seacoast.

The reason for the Finnish—and, more recently, worldwide—devotion to the sauna is that it produces many of the same physical and psychological benefits as massage. But the ideal—and few experiences are as delightful—is to follow a sauna and shower with a complete classical massage.

The Sauna Experience

If you've never taken a sauna, you'll find it a bit like stepping into a hot attic on a summer day—except that the attic might be humid. The air in the sauna is as dry as the desert, about 5 percent humidity, which means that it's rather comfortable even when the temperature is 200°F. By comparison, sitting in a tub of 100°F water would be almost intolerable for most people—and eventually fatal. A steam room would have you suffering at 140°F.

The difference is that, after about eight minutes in the sauna's dry heat, you being to perspire, and the condensation of sweat keeps the body itself cool. But you can't sweat when the air itself is moisture-laden or you're sitting in a tub of water. Only to the degree that you continue to perspire can you remain comfortable.

With sweating comes the first actual health benefits. The body's pores open widely, and the sweat that is released carries with it various impurities. Sebaceous glands excrete oil and trapped dirt. The effect is a first-class skin cleansing all over the body. That's helpful for people with skin blemishes caused by deep-seated foreign particles.

People with some forms of kidney disease may also benefit. When the kidneys are unable to flush sufficient wastes from the blood, the toxins accumulate to poison the system. Certain of these wastes can be excreted through perspiration.

That's not just theory. At Peter Bent Brigham Hospital in Boston, patients with kidney failure were put on sauna therapy for half an hour every day. Tests indicated that urea nitrogen, a waste product usually eliminated from the body through urine but which remains in the blood when the kidneys don't function properly, was excreted with the sweat of the patients in concentrations ten times that of controls. The itching that accompanies this condition was also reduced.

When people step out of the sauna, their skin is about 20 shades closer to red than when they went in—and that's evidence of another benefit. Sauna dramatically improves circulation, so that every cell of the body has a better supply of oxygen and nutrients. Intracellular wastes are flushed away so that the cells can function more efficiently. Lymph flow is increased. Heart rate and oxygen consumption rise. All in all, the effects are similar to mild exercise.

Some enthusiasts make additional health claims. They say that bacteria which cause infections can't endure high temperatures, and because a prolonged sauna raises the body temperature to about 103°F, some of these bacteria are destroyed. It's an interesting argument, but it hasn't been proven.

If you've ever had a sauna, you already know that you can walk into a sauna with problems that need decisions, and when you walk out you'll still have them, but somehow the heat has shrunk them down to size. You might go in with every muscle in your body rigid from emotional stress. Somehow, when the sweating begins, those muscles just have to relax. It's a physiological response to the heat.

Physical relaxation is probably the main reason the sauna has always been popular in Finland. A more accurate word for it is that your body feels *peace*. Tired muscles feel at ease. If you want to sleep, your body is ready for it. If after a busy day you're planning an active night, your body feels refreshed and ready to go.

During and after a sauna, the Finns traditionally beat each other with birch twigs. The practice is so old that no one knows for sure what the original intention was, but it was probably meant as a form of massage. The striking blows cause reflex contractions, and when muscles all over the body are struck, the effect is similar to a vigorous massage.

If you can arrange for your friend to take a sauna immediately before you give a massage, you'll find his or her body more receptive than usual to your efforts. The muscles will be softer and more pliant. Your friend will already be relaxed. It's like having the most strenuous part of the massage already completed. Now, because the sensitivity of the nerves is increased with improved circulation, your friend will be more aware and appreciative of your touch. You'll be able to manipulate muscle tissue more easily.

The most important guiding principle, whether you're using finger pressure or classical techniques following sauna, is that you need to be more gentle. Whether you're kneading, pressing, or striking, the muscle isn't going to resist pressure as it ordinarily would. The amount of force you usually use can now cause pain and possibly injury. A firm slide stroke that would feel good before a sauna might be painful immediately afterward. Use the same strokes, but use them gently.

On the same principle, I personally don't use oils containing eucalyptus, wintergreen, or other heat-producing substances following a sauna. For one thing, it wouldn't give any additional benefits. And of course it can be painful to the sensitized nerves. When giving classical massage, I use a plain vegetable oil as described in Chapter 2. In finger pressure massage, no lubricant should be used.

If you're not a sauna regular, make sure the temperature is not above 170°F. Experienced sauna bathers might endure temperatures of 205° (the temperature of the nail I sat on), but you're asking too much of your body to expect it to adjust to that kind of sweating requirement without conditioning.

DRESS

In the sauna, perspiration must be allowed to evaporate freely from the entire body. Saunas should be taken nude.

DURATION

The beginner should spend 7 to 10 minutes in the heat. The higher the bench, the hotter the temperature. A better guide than a stopwatch is to be sensitive to your own feelings. While you're sweating and feeling good about it, with no light-headedness, the heat is probably doing you good. But when (1) you *do* begin to feel light-headed, or (2) you've sweated so profusely that the moisture can't evaporate fast enough from your skin, making you feel uncomfortable, or (3) you're unable to sweat profusely enough to keep your core temperature moderate—leave.

The routine followed by many serious sauna bathers is this:

- From 10 to 15 minutes in the sauna
- A shower (cold, if you're a purist, lukewarm otherwise)
- A few minutes' rest
- Two more repetitions of the above cycle
- A massage

There are no obvious benefits to making three visits to the sauna instead of one, however. The important thing is to feel good and avoid extremes.

Here are some guidelines to make sauna more safe and enjoyable.

As J. J. Viherjuuri points out in his book, *Sauna, The Finnish Bath*, "A full stomach and a sauna do not agree." Wait at least an hour, preferably two, after eating before taking a sauna. Otherwise, the blood that should be in your stomach helping to digest food will be flowing to the skin to cool the body. Your stomach won't like that, and it'll let you know about it.

If you suffer from low blood pressure, consult your physician before using a sauna. Chances are, you'll get his or her blessing, but if your problem is serious, the additional drop in blood pressure which occurs as circulation increases could cause fainting.

People with heart disease should check with their physicians, too. As I've said, the heart rate increases in a sauna as it does when you exercise, and that could prove an overload for people with bad hearts. The old Department of Health, Education and Welfare once recommended labeling every sauna unit sold in the United States with a statement saying, in effect: "Warning—elderly persons or those suffering from heart disease or high or low blood pressure should not use this device unless directed by a physician."

The heavier the exercise a person engages in before going into the sauna, the less time he should spend in it. Exercise causes the body's temperature to rise, leaving a smaller safety factor before overheating occurs.

When the sauna heat is extremely dry, irritation might develop in your mucous membranes. One solution is to sprinkle a *little* water over the heated rocks to add humidity to the air. A common mistake among beginners is to pour too much water on the rocks —a 175°F steam bath is just not tolerable. Or, you can spend less time in the sauna.

Finally, be sure to remove all rings, bracelets, watches, chains, earrings, and glasses. A few minutes in the sauna and they'll become too hot to touch.

The Steam Bath

Although the Turkish, or steam, bath can be experienced in health clubs all over the country, and although it does give a physically and emotionally relaxing experience, it does not produce all the physiological benefits of the sauna. The reason is simple: It's impossible to perspire in a steam room. The major benefit of a steam bath is that it can help to break up congestion in the lungs and sinuses—but even that positive point has its negative side. Moisture-saturated air makes breathing difficult, especially if you're suffering from asthma or emphysema. People with these conditions should *not* take steam baths.

For many people, the steam bath is a singularly uncomfortable experience. Even healthy people might find it difficult to breathe. The rapid increase in temperature can also catch the inexperienced unprepared. The beginner, together with the sufferer of cardiac, respiratory, and blood pressure problems, should use extreme caution in taking a steam bath.

As a precursor to massage, steam has virtually the same effect on the muscles as the sauna. Follow the same guidelines in giving massage.

CHAPTER FOURTEEN

STRETCH EXERCISES FOR FLEXIBILITY

Many years ago, I decided to learn massage for two reasons. First, I wanted to be able to relax my friends after an emotionally stressful day. But the second reason was even more common: I wanted to have the skill to ease the pain of stiff and aching muscles, to put at ease tight shoulders, stiff necks, painful backs, and cramped legs. Those of you who through these pages have learned the art of having "good hands" will discover that most of the massages you give are aimed at relieving these same muscular problems. And in virtually all cases, these discomforts and ailments result because the muscles have grown short and stiff. That's where stretch exercises become crucial as an aid to thorough massage.

Most muscle strains are caused by a lack of flexibility. Even the most common aches and pains that doctors may diagnose as rheumatism or arthritis are often simply the result of severely limited flexibility. Calcium deposits form in joints that haven't been used throughout their full range of movement, causing an arthritic condition which may be incurable.

It needn't be that way. The conditions usually dismissed as rheumatism and arthritis can often be reversed by stretch exercises. Herbert H. DeVries, Ph.D., professor of physical education and director of the Physiology of Exercise Research Lab at the University of Southern California–Los Angeles, says, "Considerable research indicates that maintenance of good joint mobility (flexibility) prevents or to a large extent removes the aches and pains that grow more common with increasing age."

Stiff muscles can also make you feel chronically fatigued, as though everything takes too much energy. In fact, it *does*. To understand why, you must know that every skeletal muscle which creates movement is either a flexion muscle or an extension muscle. The biceps in your upper arm is a flexion muscle—it pulls the lower arm closer to the upper arm. The triceps, on the back of the arm, is an extensor muscle—it pulls the forearm outward, straightening the elbow joint.

Although the biceps and triceps (and equivalent muscle sets all over the body) work in opposition to each other, one muscle relaxes and stretches when the opposing muscle contracts. But it doesn't always work that way. Muscles that aren't used and stretched regularly shorten and lose their elasticity. Then, when its opposing muscle contracts, the contraction works not only against gravity and body weight, but against the resistance of its stiff and shortened counterpart. It really *does* require more energy to get through the day, and ordinary activities can lead to seemingly unexplainable fatigue.

Massage and Flexibility Exercise

For as long as massage has been practiced, it's been recognized as an effective way to loosen stiff muscles and keep them flexible. On a localized level, classical massage techniques manually stretch and loosen muscle fibers. What's more, muscles that are manipulated apparently respond on a neurochemical level in a way that adds another dimension to muscle relaxation. But unless massage is very vigorous and frequent—at least twice daily—it's not in itself a complete solution to chronic muscle tension.

The answer is a twice-a-week, 15-minute routine of flexibility exercises together with regular massage.

I don't mean calisthenics. Recent evidence indicates that calisthenics aren't the ideal way to develop flexibility. According to Dr. DeVries, cited earlier, "Stretching by jerking, bobbing or bouncing methods (as in calisthenics) involves the stretch reflexes, which actually oppose the desired stretching." DeVries compares calisthenics, which he calls ballistic exercises, to "static" stretching like yoga. He says, in effect, that when a muscle is jerked into extension, the natural reaction is for it to jerk back, thus shortening itself again. But when the stretch is achieved slowly and held for a period of time, another reaction takes place, the inverse myotatic reflex, which helps to relax the muscles being stretched.

DeVries gives several other advantages to static stretching:

- There is less danger of exceeding the safe limits, because the gradual increase in pain acts as a good limiting factor that prevents tight muscles from being torn when they refuse to stretch.
- Energy requirements are lower, so that a full and effective program of stretching exercises need not be exhaustive or time-consuming.
- Although ballistic stretching (calisthenics) is likely to cause muscle soreness, static stretching will not—and in fact may actually relieve sore muscles.

Do you or your friend need flexibility exercises? Muscles and joints are flexible, not people, and rare is the individual who is flexible throughout his or her body. You might be ideally flexible in most areas, but a shortened hip flexor could be subtly affecting your posture and putting a risky stress on your spine. You could have a shortened hamstring just waiting for the right excuse to give you crippling pain.

The following is a program of flexibility exercises for all the major muscles of your body. These exercises should first be used as a test. *Attempt each exercise slowly, and do not go beyond a normal degree of discomfort.* Be especially careful with exercises that put pressure on the knees, because knee injuries are common, and hard to get rid of. It's wise to bend the knees slightly if you feel tension there. Make a note of the exercises you can't accomplish, and string them together into your own flexibility program.

I promise you this: If you have short, inflexible muscles (and you can learn in 10 minutes whether you do or not), they're definitely putting a strain on your energy and vibrancy levels. You don't realize it, of course, but this is at least part of the reason you lack vitality. Use the exercises to learn which muscles are stiff, then set about stretching them for a week, and you'll feel like a rubber ball instead of a lead weight.

In putting together a flexibility program, you needn't use all of the exercises presented here—one for each stiff muscle group is sufficient. You can get by with two sessions a week. In fact, research by Dr. B. F. McCue shows that the advantages of stretching exercises can last two months or more without repetition. But you will not *improve* with that kind of schedule.

A final word: Stretching exercises have been practiced for thousands of years under the name Hatha Yoga. If you should find that you desperately need to limber up, consider buying some books or records on yoga, or sign up for a yoga class at your local YMCA. It may be one of the best investments you'll make in your overall health.

Shoulders, Neck, and Upper-Chest Stretches

EXERCISE 1

1. Interlace your fingers behind your back and, straightening your arms, lift your hands upward as far as you can. If your shoulders are flexible, you will be able to stand tall and still raise your hands to the same height as your navel.
2. Holding that position, drop your head back until the base of your skull is not more than two finger widths from your spine at the upper back.
3. Drop your head forward so that your chin rests on your chest while maintaining an upright posture, arms extended behind you.
4. While maintaining position (1) above, lower the side of your head to your shoulder. You're sufficiently flexible if your ear-lobe comes to within one finger width of touching your shoulder. (Lifting your shoulder to your ear is cheating.) Do this exercise to both left and right.

EXERCISE 2

1. Lift your left arm straight upward. Rotate it backward, downward, to the front, and finally to the starting position, keeping it straight throughout. Move at a speed that will take 2 seconds to make the entire circle, and avoid twisting your body sideward as your arm moves to the back part of the stroke.
2. Repeat with your right arm.
3. Raise both arms over your head. Sweep them back simultaneously in the same circular motion as above. When the arms move in unison, neither will reach as far back as they do individually, but your hands should be able to stretch at least 2 feet behind the plane of your shoulder for normal flexibility.

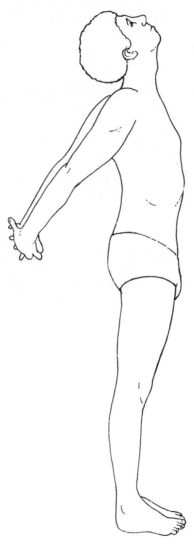

Shoulders, neck, and upper chest exercise 1. While keeping hands up and pelvis forward, drop your head back, forward, and toward each shoulder without forcing the effort.

EXERCISE 3

1. Standing in a doorway, grasp each side of the frame with hands at shoulder level.
2. Walk forward, straightening your arms behind you and standing straight. You'll feel the tug in both the chest and arm muscles. (If you're lacking in flexibility, you won't be able to stand straight while maintaining your grip and keeping your arms rigid.)

Lower-Back and Hamstring Stretch

EXERCISE 1

This actually requires flexibility in areas other than the hamstrings and lower back; you won't accomplish it if your upper back is too stiff or if your Achilles tendon has shortened. Although it's something most of us have done in grammar school, it's one of the most important flexibility exercises.

1. Sit on the floor with your legs extended, your knees slightly bent (about an inch off the floor), and your toes pointing back toward your body.
2. Lower your chin to your chest. Curl your back forward *without straining*. Stop when you feel more than minor discomfort and hold that position. Reach for your toes.
3. You have no flexibility problems in your back, hamstring, or calf muscles if you can touch your forehead to your knees while grasping your toes.

EXERCISE 2

1. Stand with your feet about a yard apart.
2. Bend at the waist and touch the floor with the palms of your hands. Don't lean so far forward that you'd fall on your face if your hands weren't there.

EXERCISE 3

1. Lie on your back with your legs straight, your arms outstretched perpendicular to your body.

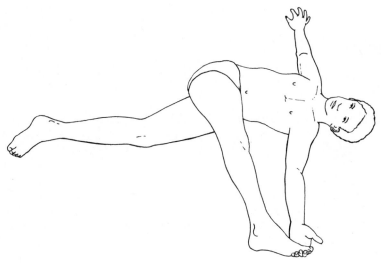

Exercise 3, the reclining toe touch.

2. Raise your right leg up to form a 90 degree angle with your
   body.
3. Bring that leg across your body and downward while your
   shoulders remain flat on the floor. Try to touch your left hand
   with your right foot.
   Repeat with your left foot.
      This exercise also stretches the gluteus medius, or muscles
   of the upper buttocks.

Calf Stretches

   Most exercises that stretch the quadriceps, or calf muscles, also
stretch the hamstrings.

EXERCISE 1

1. Standing with legs apart and your hands behind your head, twist forward and to the right until your left elbow touches your right knee.
2. Stand tall. Repeat to the left.

EXERCISE 2

1. Bend your knees and lean forward so that you support your weight on the palms of your hands and feet, including your heels.
2. Slowly straighten your knees. You'll feel the stretching in many areas—the flexor muscles of your arms, the Achilles tendon, and the gastrocnemius and quadriceps of the calves.

EXERCISE 3

1. Take one large step and another half step back from a wall.
2. Bending forward without moving your feet, place the palms of your hands flat against the wall.
3. Straighten your legs slowly, keeping your heels firmly planted.

Hip Flexor Stretches for Better Posture

Teachers from kindergarten through high school lectured us about the importance of good posture. Yet, some of us never paid attention, and today we reap the subtle harvest—nagging lower back pain, and abdomens that could launch an entire new industry—belly bras.

For most of us the problem started in childhood when we first began carrying the upper part of our bodies on an architecturally unsound foundation. Modestly, we tucked the genital region inward, rolling the buttocks out. That produced the lordotic curve at the base of the spine, subjecting the vertebrae there to continuous abnormal stress.

As that posture continued, changes took place in muscles, tendons, and ligaments, particularly the rectus femoris and quadriceps on the outside of the upper thigh. When the pelvis was tilted downward, these muscles and their tendons and ligaments shortened, and eventually this became a semipermanent condition. At that point, we no longer had an easy choice about what posture to assume. The shortened muscles forced the abnormal posture.

Here's a good way to learn if those upper thigh muscles have shortened and are forcing you into poor posture. Lie on your back on the floor with your knees bent and your pelvis tilted upward so that your entire back and buttocks are touching the floor. (If there's enough space for you to slip your hand between your spine and floor, you must rotate your pelvis more.)

Now, slowly straighten your legs while keeping your entire back against the floor. If it's impossible—if the short, tight muscles of your upper thighs force the pelvis to turn under again, arching the back—you need the following exercises.

EXERCISE 1

1. Yoga practitioners call this the *bow*. Rest on your abdomen with your legs together and your chin on the floor. Bend your knees so that your feet come up toward your head.
2. Reach back and grab your ankles firmly. Lift both your chin and your thighs off the floor so that your body takes on the appearance of an archer's bow.

EXERCISE 2

1. Take one large step away from a chair. Extend your right leg back and place your foot on the chair.
2. Bend your knee as much as necessary to hold your body erect, your pelvis rolled forward. Now, straighten your knee as much as you can without allowing your body to tilt forward.
3. Repeat with the opposite leg.

Adductor Group Stretches

If you were to ride a horse bareback as the Indians did, you'd maintain your seat by squeezing your knees tightly against the

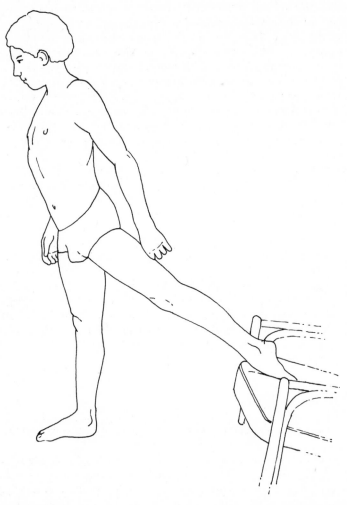

Hip flexor exercise 2 will probably be a good deal more difficult than you suspect if you do it properly. Keep both knees straight. Keep your spine straight. As you attempt to bring your upper body to a right angle with the floor, make sure you feel the strain in your upper front thigh muscles. (The tendency is to arch your back to eliminate that strain, which eliminates any benefits the exercise might bring you.)

animal's body. You'd be using the adductor muscles on the inner aspect of your upper thighs. Those are the same muscles that allow you to kick a soccer ball sideward, sweeping your leg across your body.

Relatively few of us ride horses or play soccer, however, so these muscles are likely to be short and inflexible. The following exercises will restore their elasticity—but this word of caution: The adductors are attached to the inner aspect of the knee joint, where excessive stress can cause lasting damage to ligaments. Don't try to overcome a lifetime of inflexibility in a day or two by pushing beyond mild discomfort. Repeat the exercises daily, content to progress little by little, and within a couple of weeks you'll reach your goal.

EXERCISE 1

1. Lie on your back with your legs straight and your pelvis tilted forward (your lower back against the floor). Turn the toes on your right foot outward and slide the bottom of that foot along your left leg until it rests on the left thigh above the knee.
2. Maintaining that position, lower the right knee to the floor. Keep your entire back in contact with the floor by maintaining the upward thrust of your pelvis.
3. Repeat using your opposite leg.

EXERCISE 2

1. Begin with your right foot on your left thigh as in the previous exercise. Now, raise your left foot and press it against the right one, sole to sole.
2. While tilting your pelvis forward, spread your knees to bring them closer to the floor. Keep your feet and buttocks firmly planted. Unless you're extremely flexible, your knees won't touch the floor—but you'll certainly feel the adductors stretching.

EXERCISE 3

1. Kneel in a frog position—knees as wide apart as you can manage, soles of your feet together, arms straight with palms on the floor supporting your upper body.

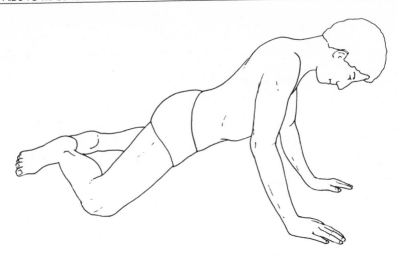

Aaductor exercise 3. Note that the feet are planted firmly together, sole to sole. That requires that the knees be spread widely. Even before you bend your arms, you'll no doubt feel the stretching along the inner part of your upper thighs—the adductors. Go slowly, and stop before you feel real pain. Going too far or too fast can cause knee injury.

2. While keeping your pelvis tilted forward, your knees and feet planted, bend your arms slightly. Proceed cautiously—you'll feel the stretching immediately.

Graduation Exercises

After you've obtained a healthy level of flexibility, there are two exercises that can help you maintain looseness in most major muscles for an investment of about one minute every three or four days. These are advanced yoga positions—to avoid injury, don't attempt them until you've mastered the previous exercises.

THE PLOUGH

1. Lie on your back with your arms at your sides, palms down on the floor. Keeping your legs *straight*, raise them over your head so that your toes touch the floor above your head.

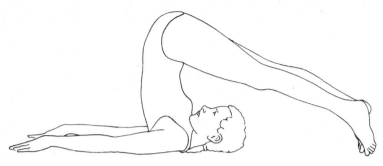

The plough.

2. Bend your knees, making them touch the floor on either side of your head.

THE ADVANCED CAMEL

1. Start in a kneeling position, grasping your ankles. Very *slowly*, lower your body back until your head touches the floor. If you can't stretch the upper thigh muscles sufficiently, release your ankles and use your hands to support your body weight at whatever angle you're able to reach.
2. Tilt your pelvis forward, arching your abdomen and dropping your head back.
3. The ultimate achievement is to rest with your head on the floor, hands on your ankles, buttocks not touching your heels, and abdomen arched upward.

CONCLUSION

When I was a boy, I had an English teacher named Mr. Wilkes. At the time, I hated to read, and as a result, I hated to do the book reports Mr. Wilkes (and the English teachers who had preceded him) required. One morning when the class was in the library choosing books for the next book report and I was hunting for the smallest book with the largest pictures that I could find, I felt a large hand on my shoulder. Mr. Wilkes, who had recognized that I was a tense, hyperactive child, gently massaged my shoulder and neck. It lasted for only a few seconds, but it was long enough to make me feel special and cared about.

Then Mr. Wilkes pulled a book from the shelf: *The Black Stallion*. It was a massive tome, more than 200 pages. "I want you to read this book," he said, handing it to me. I thought it would take a lifetime to get through it, but Mr. Wilkes had shown me that he thought I was special, and I did not want to disappoint him. I read it in three days. In the next few months I read a dozen more books; later, I began writing books of my own, although the first was not published until I was 20.

I owe a career to the touch of a single hand.

A few years ago, a friend of mine named Myra was deeply in love with a young doctor. They were engaged to be married and the date was set. At his insistance, she gave up her job, shopped for an apartment, and began planning to decorate it. Then, the doctor met an old girl friend, began dating her, and eventually cancelled the wedding plans with Myra. On the verge of an emotional breakdown, Myra went to see her family doctor.

Dr. Dry was in his late sixties by then. He was from the old school and felt that the people who walked into his office were not merely patients but also people. He'd often walk into the treatment room with the question, "What's happening in your life lately?" And you knew he really wanted to know.

As Myra began to answer, he moved behind her and placed both of his hands on her shoulders. As he gently massaged the stiff muscles, she began to cry. He kept massaging and for a long while she kept crying.

"Do you want to talk about it?" he asked when she'd grown silent. She shook her head.

"I don't have to talk about it now. I'll be all right. Thank you."

In the security of Dr. Dry's two hands, Myra felt safe enough to release her pain.

At age 34, Charlotte Snow, my wife's sister, was dying of liver cancer in a York, Pennsylvania, hospital. We were alone in her room. She shuddered in pain. The sweat glistened on her face. Her eyes were filled with fear.

"I don't want to die," she told me.

I sat beside her on the bed and took her hands in mine. I caressed each finger, the backs of her hands, the palms, her arms. After a few minutes she smiled and closed her eyes and slept peacefully until the end came.

If there is any gift among humankind more potent and precious than the gift of good hands, hands that can convey compassion, I don't know about it. Jesus exercised it. The finest physicians from ancient China and classical Greece, of all nations and all times including our own, understood the power in their hands.

In these pages I've given you the fundamentals, the knowledge to work with. That was the easy part. And to tell you the truth, it's the smallest part.

After all is said and done, good hands come from the heart.

ADDITIONAL READINGS

Paul Becker and Elizabeth C. Wood. *Beard's Massage*. Philadelphia, Pa.: W. B. Saunders, 1981.

Ann H. Downer, *Physical Therapy Procedures*, 3rd ed. Springfield, III: Charles C. Thomas, 1975.

Maria Ebner, *Connective Tissue Massage*. Melbourne, Fla.: Krieger, 1977.

Bonnie Prudden, *Pain Erasure*, New York: M. Evans & Co., 1980.

Manipulation, Traction and Massage, 2nd. ed. Joseph B. Rogoff, M. D. (ed.), Baltimore, Md.: Williams & Wilkins, 1980.

Frances M. Tappan, *Healing Massage Techniques*. Reston, Va.: Reston, 1978.

Frederick Leboyer, *Loving Hands: The Traditional Indian Art of Baby Massaging*, New York: Knopf, 1976.

Watari Ohashi, *Do-It-Yourself Shiatsu*, Unwin Paperbacks, 1979.

H. J. Viherjuuri, *Sauna: The Finnish Bath*, Brattleboro, Vt.: Greene, 1965.

Gordon Inkeles, *The New Massage: Total Body Conditioning for People Who Exercise*, Unwin Paperbacks, 1981.

Other recommended reading . . .

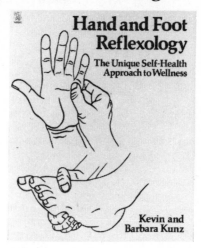

Hand and Foot Reflexology

- Why your feet and hands are important sensory organs, and their special relationship with your whole body
- Why reflexology works
- Specially designed pressure and movement techniques that reduce stress and actually alter the body's tension level
- Fully illustrated, with step-by-step procedures for quick and easy application
- Treatment plans for specific ailments
- 'Stride Replication', the authors' latest programme of foot and hand relaxation

Here's a revolutionary way to fine-tune your relationship with your body, reduce stress and feel better all over: stimulate the reflexes in your hands and feet!

It's all in this hands-on encyclopaedia of personal reflexology information. Here, Kevin and Barbara Kunz (authors of *The Complete Guide to Foot Reflexology*) bring you their unique *self-health approach to wellness*. Through reflexology they teach you how to free and channel your pent-up energy — and to prevent and correct common health problems.

Whether you use it as a quick reference or as the basis for further study this book tells you what you need to know about the simple but potent experience of reflexology — by yourself and for yourself.